방사선사를 위한

병원실무영어

HOSPITAL PRACTICAL ENGLISH FOR THE RADIOLOGICAL TECHNOLOGIST

유광열 · 이주영

도서출판 대학서림

PREFACE

우리는 현재 국제화 시대에 발맞추어 다문화 가정이 크게 확산되고 있고, 앞으로 해외 취업을 원하는 학생들도 크게 늘어나고 있는 상황이며, 의료분야의 최고를 자랑하는 우리나라는 외국인들의 의료 수요가 급격히 증가되고 있습니다. 의료기관 특히 방사선 진료 업무 분야도 예외 없이 국제화를 위해 모든 업무가 국제 표준을 따르도록 많은 노력을 기울이고 있습니다. 의료기관을 방문하는 환자들을 직접 상대해야 하는 방사선사들에게 있어서 보다 나은 진료 서비스를 베풀어야 하는 일은 너무나 당연한 일이며, 특히 외국인의 경우에도 예외가 될 수 없을 것입니다. 이를 위해서는 최우선적으로 원만한 의사소통이 전제되어야 할 것입니다. 올바른 의사소통이 이루어지지 않는다면 아무리 훌륭한 진료 서비스가 이루어진다고 하여도 올바른 진료성과를 거둘 수 없을 것입니다. 이 책은 방사선사로서 실무에서 자주 부딪히게 되는 현장의 상황을 가정하여 실제 업무에 직접 사용할 수 있도록 가능한 한 쉬운 표현으로 대화를 구성하였습니다.

특히 이 책은 방사선학을 전공하는 학생들이 대학에서 현장 영어를 익히고 실무에서 사용할 수 있도록 구성하였고, 일반 촬영을 비롯한 영상의학 분야와 방사선종양학, 핵의학 분야 등의 각 방사선분야 별로 나누어 실무와 관련된 영어회화 수업의 교과목에 활용할 수 있도록 하였습니다. 더불어 방사선 분야 취업을 위한 인터뷰의 사례를 실었습니다. 이 책에 나오는 일부 대화내용과 사진들은 이미 널리 공개된 내용에서 발췌된 내용을 중심으로 인용, 편집하였음을 알려드립니다.

2024년 2월 편저자

CONTENTS

방사선사를 위한 **병원실무영어**

Chapter 1.1
진료예약하기

A Dialogue

SITUATION ❶ I would like to schedule a doctor's appointment.

Receptionist Hello, this is Hankook Hospital. How may I assist you?

Patient I'd like to schedule an appointment to see a doctor.

Receptionist Certainly. What's the reason for your appointment?

Patient I've been experiencing a stomachache all day.

Receptionist Thank you. Have you visited us before?

Patient No, it's my first time.

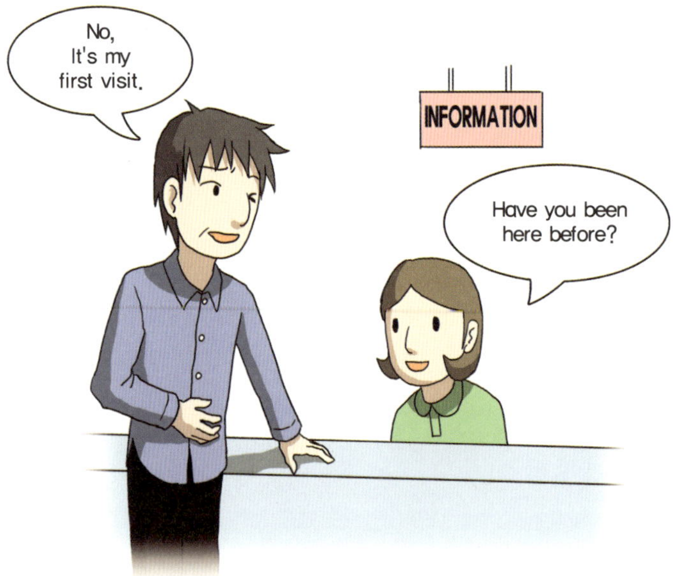

No,
It's my
first visit.
INFORMATION
Have you been
here before?

Receptionist	Sure. May I have your name, please?
Patient	Mason Jones.
Receptionist	Thank you. What's your date of birth?
Patient	January 16, 1978.
Receptionist	And your cell phone number?"

SITUATION ❷ Let me check for an available time.

Receptionist Let me check for an available time. The earliest one is tomorrow morning at 10:30 a.m. Will that work for you?

Patient Is 11 a.m. available instead of 10:30 a.m. on the same day?

Receptionist Unfortunately, 11 a.m. is already booked, but we do have an opening at 11:30 a.m. Is that suitable for you?

Patient That works for me. I'll take it.

Receptionist Great! I've scheduled your appointment for 11:30 on Wednesday morning.

Patient Thank you very much.

Receptionist You're welcome. If you need to reschedule, please call us at 031-321-5231 with 24 hours' notice. Is there anything else I can assist you with?

Patient No, that's all. Thank you for your help. Have a good day!

Receptionist You're welcome, sir. Have a wonderful day!

* make an appointment to see a doctor : 진료예약을 하다.
* instead of : ~대신에, * in advance : 미리, 사전에

B Reviewing Useful Expressions

1 I want to schedule a doctor's appointment

2 What's the reason for the appointment?

3 Have you visited us before?

4 Let me check for an available time.

5 If you need to reschedule your appointment, please call us ahead of time.

C Role playing

진료 예약하기 ❶

접수　한국병원입니다. 무엇을 도와드릴까요?

환자　진료예약을 하려고 합니다.

접수　예, 어떻게 예약을 해드릴까요?

환자　제가 하루 종일 복통으로 시달렸어요.

접수　알겠습니다. 우리 병원이 처음이신가요?

환자　예. 처음입니다.

접수　알겠습니다. 성함이 어떻게 되시나요?

환자　Mason Jones입니다.

접수 생년월일이 어떻게 되시나요?

환자 1978년 1월 16일입니다.

접수 휴대폰 번호는 어떻게 되시나요?

진료 예약하기 ❷

접수 진료가 가능한 예약일정을 확인해 보겠습니다. 가장 빠른 예약은 내일 오전 10시 30분입니다. 그 시간이면 환자분은 괜찮으신가요?

환자 같은 날로 10시 30분 대신에 11시에는 예약이 있나요?

접수 잠깐만요, 11시에는 이미 예약이 차 있습니다. 11시 30분에는 예약이 가능합니다. 그 시간이면 괜찮으신가요?

환자 좋습니다. 그 시간으로 하겠습니다.

접수 수요일 아침 11:30으로 예약해 두겠습니다.

환자 감사합니다.

접수 천만에요. 만일 예약을 변경 하시려면, 미리 24시간 전에 전화 031-321- 5231로 연락을 주세요. 제가 도와 드릴 일이 또 있으신가요?

환자 이제는 없습니다. 도와주셔서 감사합니다. 좋은 하루 되세요.

접수 천만에요, 좋은 하루 되세요.

D Quiz

1 What's the reason for the (   )?

2 Let me check for an (   ) time.

3 That works for me. I'll (   ) it.

4 Please call us at 031-321-5231 with 24 hours' (   ).

정답 appointment / available / take / notice

E Translate Korean into English

1 한국병원입니다. 무엇을 도와드릴까요?

2 우리 병원이 처음이신가요?

3 진료가 가능한 예약일정을 확인해 보겠습니다.

4 11시에는 이미 예약이 차 있습니다. 11시 30분에는 예약이 가능합니다.

TIP! **MAKE**

- **만들다. 제작하다.** I made him a new suit.(=I made a new suit for him.)
- **~이 되다.** One and two makes three.
- **준비하다.** make a bed 잠자리를 준비하다. / make a dinner 저녁 준비를 하다.
- **해내다.** I made it! (잘 해냈다!) / I'd like to make an appointment to see a doctor.
- **획득하다. 얻다.** She makes lots of money aon the deal. (그녀는 거래를 통해 많은 돈을 벌었다.)

Chapter 1.2
진료하기

A Dialogue

SITUATION ❶ What's bothering you today?

Doctor Good morning. What's bothering you today?

Patient I'm feeling really sick, and I've been vomiting.

Doctor When did this start?

Patient It started last night, and I haven't slept well.

Doctor Any other symptoms?

Patient I also feel nauseous.

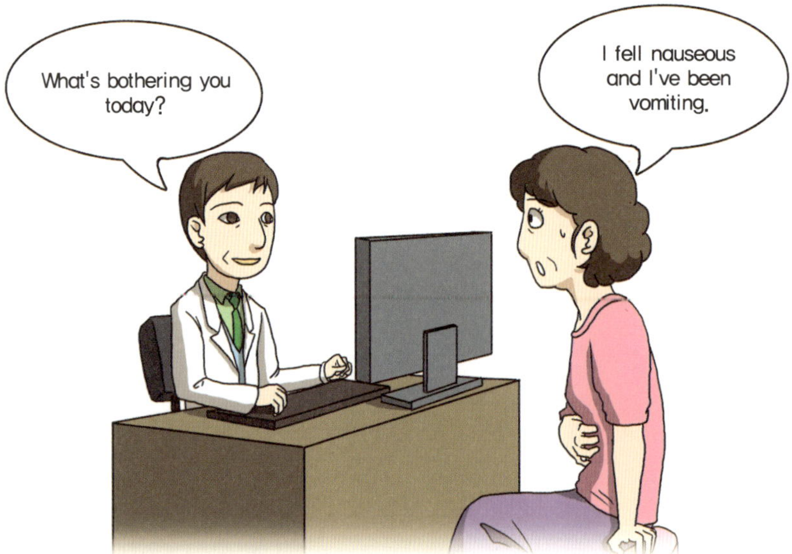
What's bothering you today?
I fell nauseous and I've been vomiting.

Doctor What did you have for dinner last night?

Patient I had seafood.

Doctor It's possible the seafood wasn't good. How's your digestion?

Patient No issues there. I don't have diarrhea, but my stomach feels bloated.

Doctor You might have a mild case of food poisoning. I'll prescribe some medication for you.

* describe : 설명하다, * symptom : 증상, * nauseous : 메스꺼운, * diarrhea : 설사, * prescribe : 처방하다, * feels bloated : 팽만감을 느끼다, *medicine : 약, * food poisoning : 식중독

B Reviewing Useful Expressions

1 What's bothering you today?

2 When did your symptoms start?

3 What did you have for dinner last night?

4 You might have a mild case of food poisoning.

5 I'll prescribe some medication for you.

C Role playing

의사 안녕하세요. 어디가 아프신가요?

환자 몸이 좋지 않습니다. 토했어요.

의사 언제 그런 증상이 시작됐나요?

환자 지난밤에요. 잠도 잘 못잤어요.

의사 그 외에, 다른 증상이 있나요?

환자 매스꺼운 느낌도 들어요.

의사 지난 밤에 무엇을 드셨나요?

환자 해산물을 먹었어요.

의사 아마 해산물이 상했나 봅니다. 장운동은 어떤가요?

환자 장에는 이상이 없는 것 같습니다. 설사도 없고요. 그런데 위장이 더부룩합니다.

의사 환자분은 경미한 식중독인 것 같습니다. 약을 처방해 드리겠습니다.

D Quiz

1 What's (   ) you today?

2 When did your (   ) start?

3 I'm feeling really sick. I've been (   ).

4 My stomach feels (   ).

정답 bothering / symptoms / vomiting / bloated

E Translate Korean into English

1 어디가 아프신가요?

2 증상을 말해보실까요?

3 설사도 하셨나요?

4 약을 처방해 드리겠습니다.

TIP! have

❶ **가지다, 소유하다.** I have a problem.
❷ **~있다, ~없다.** Do you have any other symptoms? There are a lot of people. (저 쪽에는 사람이 많다.)
❸ **시키다.** I had my photograph taken. (나는 사진을 찍었다.)
❹ **먹다, 마시다.** I had seafood and rice.
❺ **~을 하다.** have a bath(목욕하다.) / have a chat(잡담하다.) / have a drink(한잔하다.) / have a rest(잠깐 쉬다.) / have a try(한번 해보다.)

통 증

headache : 두통 / sore throat : 인후통 / back pain : 요통 / fever : 발열
chest pain : 흉통 / toothache : 치통 / runny nose : 콧물 / stomachache : 복통
menstrual pain : 생리통 / muscular pain : 근육통

Chapter 2.1

진료부서 찾기와 검사 예약하기

A Dialogue

SITUATION ❶ Could you direct me to the Radiology department?

Patient: Hi, I think I'm a bit lost. Can you tell me where the Surgery Department is?

Receptionist: "Of course, it's on the 2nd floor of this building. Just take the elevator, turn right, and you'll see the sign for the Surgery Department. It's right next to the operating room. Is there anything else I can assist you with?

Patient: Yes, I also need to get an X-ray. Could you please direct me to the Radiology Department?

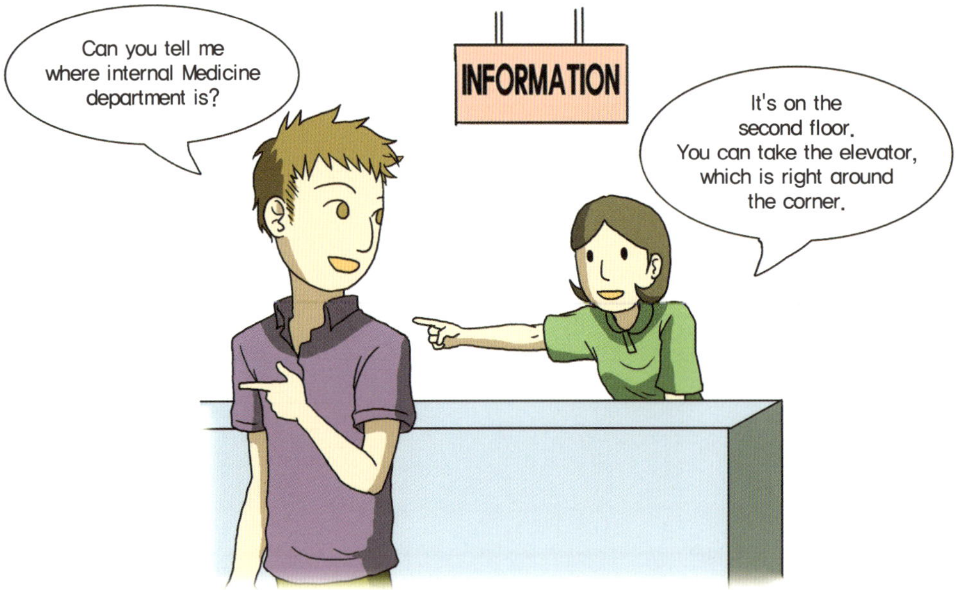
Can you tell me
where internal Medicine
department is?
INFORMATION
It's on the
second floor.
You can take the elevator,
which is right around
the corner.

Receptionist Sure, it's on the first floor of the east wing. We're currently in the south wing. Just continue straight down this hallway, and when you reach the pharmacy, take a left. You'll find the Radiology Department's reception area there.

Patient Thank you.

B Reviewing Useful Expressions

1 It's on the second floor. Just take the elevator.

2 It's on the first floor of the east wing.

3 Just continue straight down this hallway, and when you reach the pharmacy, take a left.

C Role playing

환자 안녕하세요. 제가 길을 잃은 것 같군요. 외과가 있는 곳을 알려주시겠어요?

직원 예. 외과는 이 건물 2층에 있습니다. 환자분께서는 엘리베이터를 타신 다음, 오른쪽으로 돌아가시면 외과 안내표지판을 찾으실 수 있을 겁니다. 수술실 옆입니다. 또 다른 궁금한 것이라도 있으신가요?

환자 예, 저는 또 X선 검사를 받아야 합니다. 방사선과가 어디에 있는지 알려주시겠어요?

직원 그 곳은 동관 1층에 있는데요, 여기는 서관입니다. 이 복도를 따라 곧장 가시다가 약국이 나오면 외쪽으로 돌아가세요. 그러면 방사선과 접수창구가 보일 겁니다.

환자 감사합니다.

D Quiz

1 Can you tell me (   ) the Surgery Department is?

2 It's on the 2nd floor. Just (   ) the elevator.

3 I also need to (   ) a X-ray.

4 Just continue straight down this hallway, and (   ) you reach the pharmacy, take a left.

정답 when / get / take / where

E Translate Korean into English

1 제가 길을 잃은 것 같군요. 외과가 있는 곳을 알려주시겠어요?

2 외과는 이 건물 2층에 있습니다.

3 환자분께서는 엘리베이터를 타신 다음, 오른쪽으로 돌아가시면 외과 안내표지판을 찾으실 수 있을 겁니다.

4 그 곳은 동관 1층에 있는데요, 여기는 서관입니다.

TIP! go

1. **가다.** I'm going home.
2. **진행되다.** Go on! (계속 해!)
3. **생기다.** It goes like this. (그건 이렇게 생겼어.)

TIP! directions

1. 복도를 가다가 오른쪽으로 가세요. Follow this hall, then turn right.
2. 계단을 이용하세요. Take the stairs , please.
3. 한 층 더 올라가세요. Go up one more floor
4. 두 층 더 내려가세요. Go down two more floors.
5. X선 촬영실이 나올 때까지 이 복도를 따라 계속 가세요. Keep going down this hallway until you reach the X-ray room.
6. 검사실 앞에 있습니다. It is in front of exam room. (뒤 behind / 모퉁이 at the corner / 대각선 방향 caddy corner from / 건너편 across from)

병원 진료부서(Hospital Departments)

응급실 : Emergency Room (ER)
안내 : Information Desk
접수 : Reception Desk
집중치료실 : Intensive Care Unit (ICU)
건강검진 : Medical Check-up Center
중앙검사실 : Central Laboratory
영상의학과(진단방사선과) : Radiology Department
영안실 : Mortuary
분만실 : Delivery Room
수술실 : Operating Room (OR)
마취과 : Anesthesiology
약국 : Pharmacy/Dispensary
내과 : Internal Medicine

소화기내과 : Gastroenterology
신경과 : Neurology
정신과 : Psychiatry
외과 : Surgery
정형외과 : Orthopedic Surgery
성형외과 : Plastic Surgery
산부인과 : Obstetrics and Gynecology
소아과 : Pediatrics
피부과 : Dermatology
비뇨기과 : Urology
이비인후과 : ENT
안과 : Ophthalmology
치과 : Dentistry

Chapter 2.2

검사를 접수하고 예약하기

A Dialogue

SITUATION 1 Let me check the computer quickly

Receptionist Good morning, how can I assist you?

Patient Yes, I'm Emma Williams, and my doctor referred me here.

Receptionist Let me check the computer quickly.

Patient Sure.

Receptionist I see here that you're Emma Williams, and you're scheduled for a chest X-ray, both PA and Lateral.

Patient Yes, that's correct.

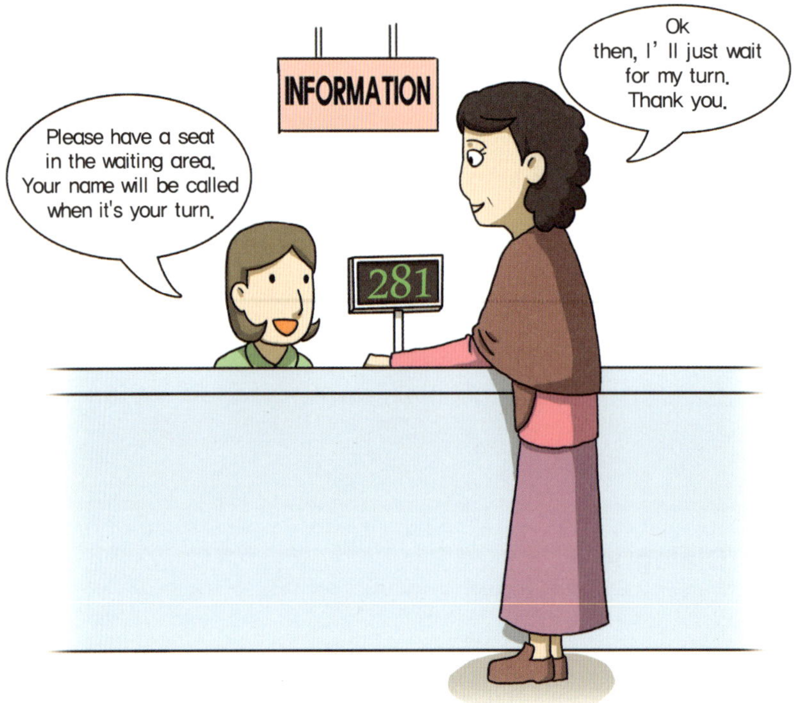

Receptionist	Please have a seat in the waiting area. Your name will be called when it's your turn. There are a few patients ahead of you.
Patient	How many patients are ahead of me?
Receptionist	There are about three patients ahead of you.
Patient	Alright, I'll wait for my turn. Thank you.
Receptionist	You're welcome, ma'am.

B Reviewing Useful Expressions

1 How can I assist you?

2 You're scheduled for a chest x-ray.

3 Your name will be called when it's your turn.

4 There are a few patients ahead of you.

5 I'll wait for my turn.

C Role playing

접수 안녕하세요. 무엇을 도와드릴까요?

환자 예, 제 이름은 Emma Williams이고요, 제 의사 선생님이 의뢰하신 검사를 하러 왔어요.

접수 먼저 컴퓨터로 조회를 해 보겠습니다.

환자 예.

접수 환자분 성함이 Emma Williams이시구요, 흉부 PA와 측면촬영을 하시는 군요.

환자 예 맞습니다.

접수 저희가 환자분 이름을 부를 때 까지 대기실에서 기다려주세요. 환자분 앞서 오신 분들이 몇 분이 계십니다.

환자 제 앞에 몇 명의 환자가 있나요?

접수 약 3명의 환자가 있습니다.

환자 예, 그럼 제 차례를 기다리겠습니다. 고맙습니다.

접수 천만에요.

D Quiz

1 Let me check the computer (   ).

2 Your name will be (   ) when it's your turn.

3 How many patients are (   ) of me?

4 I'll wait for my (   ).

정답 turn / ahead / called / quickly

E Translate Korean into English

1 먼저 컴퓨터로 조회를 해 보겠습니다.

2 환자분 성함이 Emma Williams이시구요, 흉부 PA와 측면촬영을 하시는 군요.

3 저희가 환자분 이름을 부를 때까지 대기실에서 기다려주세요.

TIP! may

❶ **~해도 좋다.** We may call her a good radiotechnologist.
❷ **~하시오.** You may go now. (지금 가도 좋습니다.)
❸ **~일지 모른다.** I'm afraid it may rain tomorrow. (내일 비가 올지 모른다.)
❹ **기원, 희망** May you be healthy. (건강하시길 빕니다.)

Chapter 3
흉부 검사하기

A Dialogue

SITUATION ❶ Please remove your bra and necklace as metal can show up on X-rays.

Radiographer	Patient Emma Williams... Is Emma Williams here?
Patient	That's me. I'm here.
Radiographer	Are you Emma Williams?
Patient	Yes, I am.
Radiographer	Alright, ma'am. Please proceed to the dressing room, change your blouse, and put on a hospital gown. Remove your bra and necklace since metal objects can be seen on X-rays.
Patient	Do I need to undress my lower body?
Radiographer	No, that's not necessary. Just tie up your hair. We have extra hair ties if you need one.

* hairclip : 머리핀, * metal object : 금속물질, * fasten : 묶다.

SITUATION ❷

Radiographer Alright, please follow me, ma'am, and I'll take your X-ray. I'll give you some instructions to follow.

Patient Okay, sure.

Radiographer Okay, ma'am, please stand straight facing the X -ray board. Lean your chest against it. Rest your chin here. Put your hands on your hips with your palms facing out.

Patient Like this?

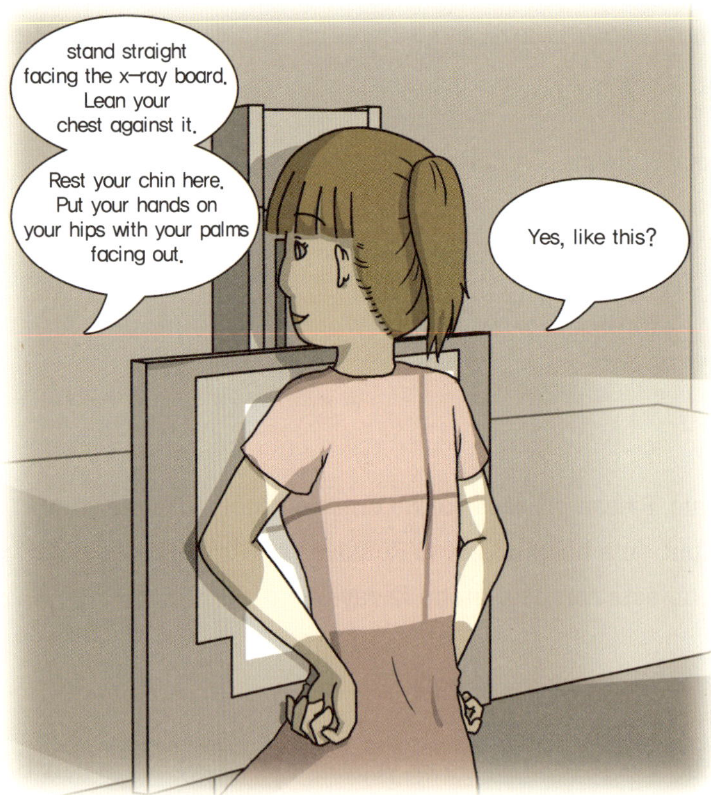

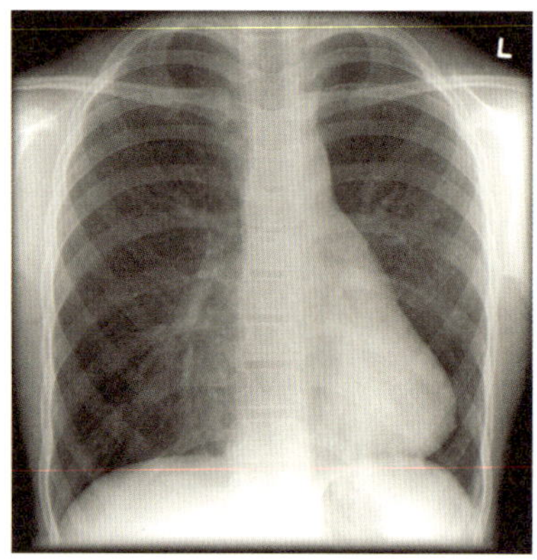

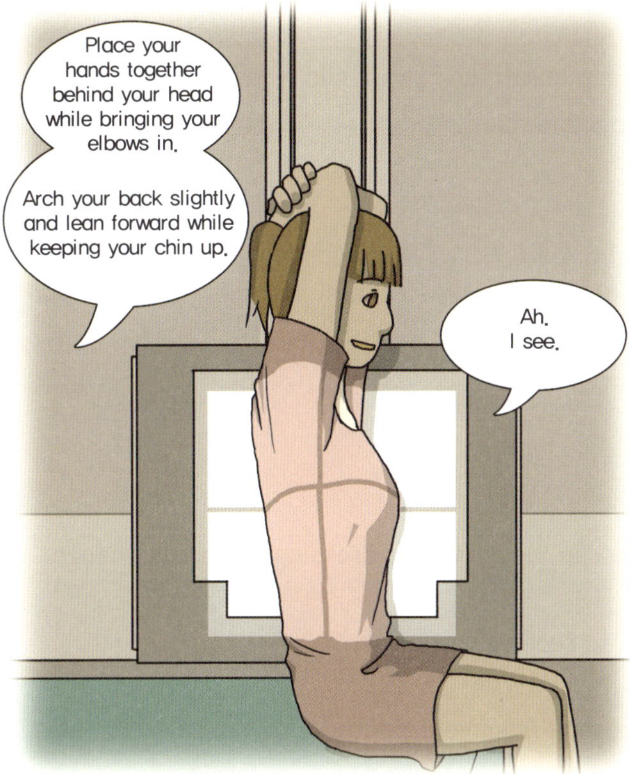

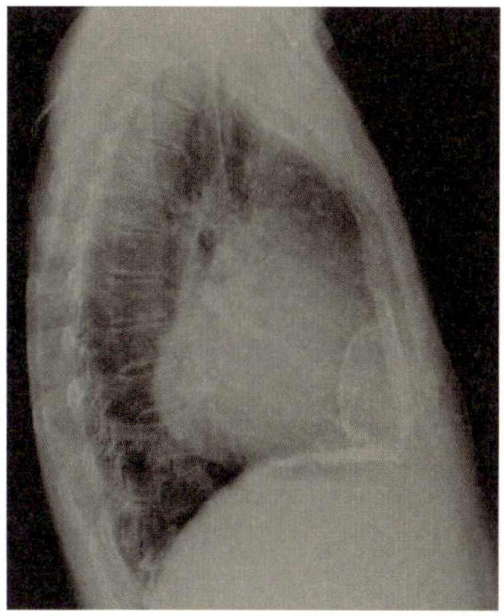

Radiographer Yes, ma'am. Please remain still. Take a deep breath and hold it... hold your breath. (click!) Alright, ma'am, you can breathe now and relax.

Patient Are we finished?

Radiographer Not yet, ma'am. We need to take the lateral view of your chest.

Patient Okay, what should I do?

Radiographer Ma'am, please turn to the side. Place your hands together behind your head while bringing your elbows in. Arch your back slightly and lean forward while keeping your chin up.

Patient Ah, I understand now.

Radiographer Hold still. Take a deep breath and then hold it (click!) Alright, ma'am, you can breathe now and relax.

* instruction : 지침, 지시, * stand straight : 똑바로 서다., * lean : 기대서다., * rest : 쉬다, 받혀놓다., * wrap : 감싸다., * take a deep breath : 심호흡하다., * hold a breath : 숨을 멈추다., * clasp : 감싸안다.

SITUATION ❸

Radiographer We're finished. You can return to the dressing room and change.

Patient When can I expect to receive the results?

Radiographer You can get your results from your doctor.

Patient Thank you.

Radiographer You're welcome, ma'am.

B Reviewing Useful Expressions

1 Please proceed to the dressing room, change your blouse, and put on a hospital gown.

2 I'll give you some instructions to follow.

3 Remove your bra and necklace since metal objects can be seen on X-rays.

4 Stand straight facing the x-ray board. Lean your chest against it.

5 Put your hands on your hips with your palms facing out.

6 Place your hands together behind your head while bringing your elbows in.

7 Please remain still. Take a deep breath and hold it.

8 We need to take the lateral view of your chest.

9 You can return to the dressing room and change.

C Role playing

상황 ❶

방사선사 여기 Emma Williams님 계시나요?

환자 제 이름이군요. 저 여기 있습니다.

방사선사 당신이 Emma Williams이신가요?

환자 예, 접니다.

방사선사 예 환자분, 탈의실에 가셔서 상의를 벗고 병원 가운으로 갈아입으세요. 금속물질은 X선 사진에 나오니 브라와 목걸이도 제거하여 주세요.

환자 알겠습니다. 하의도 벗어야 하나요?

방사선사 하의는 벗지 않아도 됩니다. 그리고 머리카락은 머리위로 올려주시고 머리끈으로 묶어 주세요. 머리끈이 없으시면 이 머리끈으로 묶어주세요.

(환자가 옷을 갈아입고 탈의실에서 나온다.)

상황 ❷

방사선사　환자분. 이쪽으로 오세요. X선 촬영을 하겠습니다. 몇 가지 환자분이 따라 해주셔야 할 지시사항을 알려드리겠습니다.

환자　예 알겠습니다.

방사선사　좋습니다. 환자분, 촬영판을 대고 똑바로 선 다음 가슴을 기대세요. 턱은 촬영판 위에 놓으세요. 손은 주먹을 쥐고 엉덩이 위에 놓으세요. 그리고 팔로 촬영판을 감아 안으세요.

환자　예, 이렇게요?

방사선사　예 환자분. 움직이지 마세요. 숨을 깊이 들어 마시고 그대로 참으세요.
(방사선사가 X선을 조사한다. 찰칵!)
좋습니다. 이제 숨을 쉬시고 편하게 계세요.

환자　끝났나요?

방사선사　이직 끝나지 않았습니다. 다른 촬영이 있는데 측면상 사진입니다.

환자　좋아요, 제가 어떻게 해야 하나요?

방사선사　환자분 이쪽을 향해주십시오. 이 옆면으로요. 팔을 올리시고 두 손은 머리 뒤로 감싸고 팔꿈치는 안쪽으로 모으세요. 등을 똑바로 펴시고 앞쪽으로 조금 숙여주세요. 턱은 올려주세요.

환자　예 알겠습니다.

방사선사　움직이지 마세요. 그대로 서 계시고. 숨을 깊게 들여 마시고 그대로 참으세요. (방사선사가 X선을 조사한다. 찰칵!)
좋습니다. 환자분. 이제 숨을 쉬어도 됩니다. 편하게 계세요.

상황 ❸

방사선사　검사가 모두 끝났습니다. 탈의실로 가셔서 옷을 갈아입도록 하세요.

환자　그런데 언제 결과를 알 수 있나요?

방사선사　결과는 재진 시 환자분의 담당 의사에게 알아보시면 됩니다.

환자　감사합니다.

방사선사　천만에요.

D Quiz

1 Please proceed to the dressing room, change your blouse, and ( ) on a hospital gown.

2 Remove your bra and necklace since ( ) can be seen on X-rays.

3 I'll ( ) you some instructions to follow.

4 Put your hands on your ( ) with your ( ) facing out.

5 ( ) a deep breath and hold it.

6 Place your ( ) together behind your head while bringing your ( ) in.

정답 put / metal objects / give / hips / palms / take / hands / elbows

E Translate Korean into English

1 환자분, 탈의실에 가셔서 상의를 벗고 병원 가운으로 갈아입으세요.

2 금속물질은 X선 사진에 나오니 브라와 목걸이도 제거하여 주세요.

3 머리카락은 머리위로 올려주시고 머리끈으로 묶어 주세요.

4 촬영판을 대고 똑바로 선 다음 가슴을 기대세요. 턱은 촬영판 위에 놓으세요.

5 움직이지 마세요. 그대로 서 계시고, 숨을 깊게 들여 마시고 그대로 참으세요.

6 팔을 올리시고 두 손은 머리 뒤로 감싸고 팔꿈치는 안쪽으로 모으세요.

TIP! keep

❶ **한 상태로 계속 유지하다.** Let's keep in touch(연락하고 지내요.)
❷ **간직하다.** keep the change. (거스름 돈 가지세요.)
❸ **이행하다.** I always keep my word. (언제나 약속을 지킨다.)
❹ **적어놓다.** keep a dairy. (일기를 쓰다.)
❺ **축하하다.** keep a Christmas. (크리스마스를 축하하다.)

TIP! keep ↔ let

keep : 활동성 있는 것, 변환 가능성이 있는 것을 원래대로 유지하도록 한다.
let : 유지시키던 것을 활동 변화가 가능 하도록 놓아준다.
keep away. (가까이 오지마.)
keep it in (숨을 참고) ↔ let it out (숨을 쉬라.)
keep it out ↔ let it in / keep it up ↔ let it down /
keep it down ↔ let it up

Chapter 4

무릎 뼈 검사하기

A Dialogue

SITUATION ❶ Position one of your legs out in front of you and slightly bend your knees.

Radiographer	Patient William Davis.
Patient	I'm here.
Radiographer	You've requested knee AP and lateral X-rays.
Patient	What does that involve?
Radiographer	We'll take two images, one from the front and one from the side, to get a complete picture of your knees. So, you'll have two X-rays done.
Patient	Is it safe? I'll be exposed to radiation twice.
Radiographer	Don't worry, sir. The radiation dose is very low, and your doctor needs the X-rays to diagnose any potential issues with your knee bones.

Patient　Ah, I see. I understand now.

Radiographer　Sir, please head to the dressing room, change your clothes, and put on the hospital gown.

Patient　Should I take off my pants?

Radiographer　Yes, sir, please remove your pants and then wear a hospital gown.

Patient　Okay, I'll do that.

* AP(anteroposterior) : 전후 방향의, 전면촬영자세, * lateral : 측면의, * dose : X선의 선량,
* dangerous : 위험한, * negligible : 무시할 수 있는

SITUATION ❷

Radiographer　Please lie down on the examination table.

Patient　Right here?

Radiographer　Yes, sir. Lie down straight while I place the board under your legs. Try to remain still.

Radiographer　Sir, please turn to your side. I'll be taking the side view. Position one of your legs out in front of the other and slightly bend your knees.

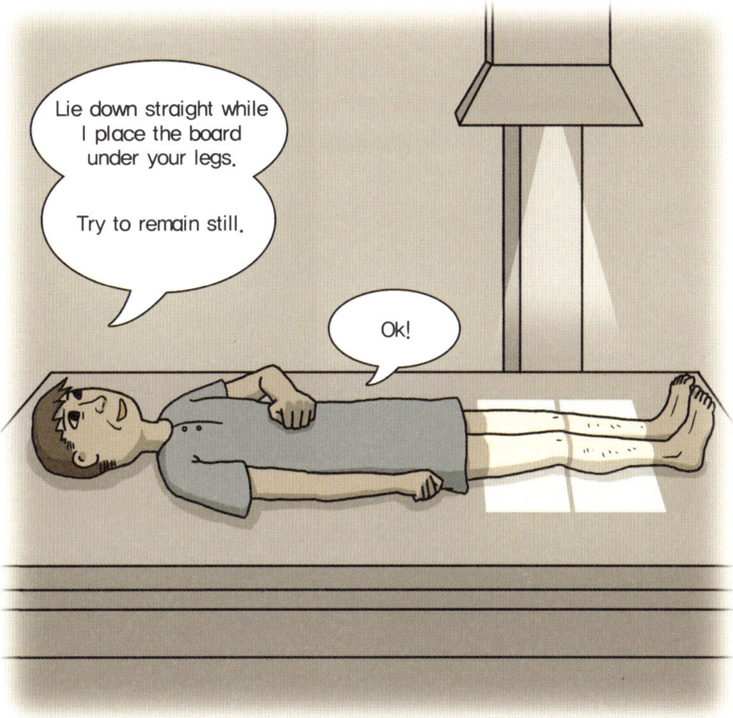

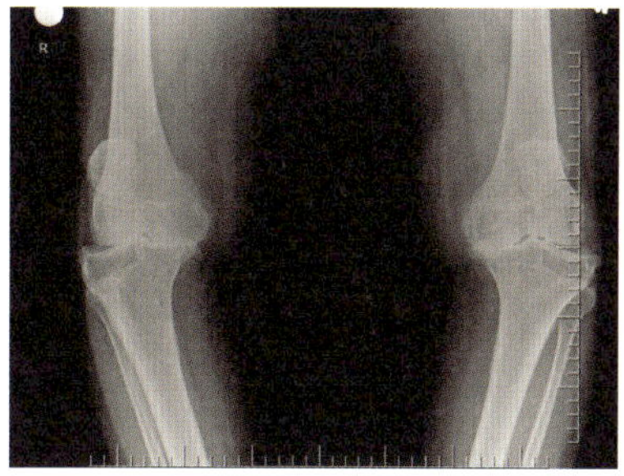

Patient I understand, like this?

Radiographer That's perfect. Please remain still while I take the X-ray.

Patient Okay.

Radiographer The examination is finished. You can now get up and change in the dressing room.

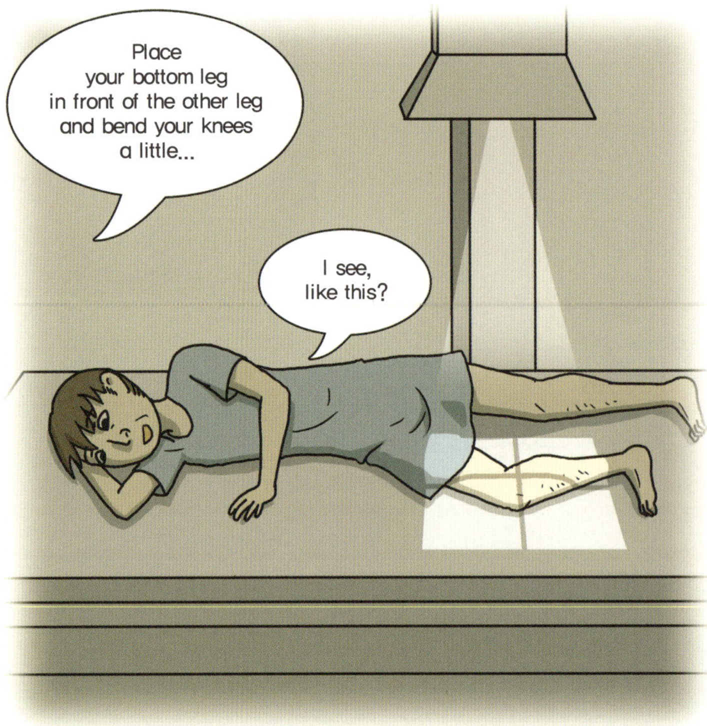
Place your bottom leg in front of the other leg and bend your knees a little...
I see, like this?

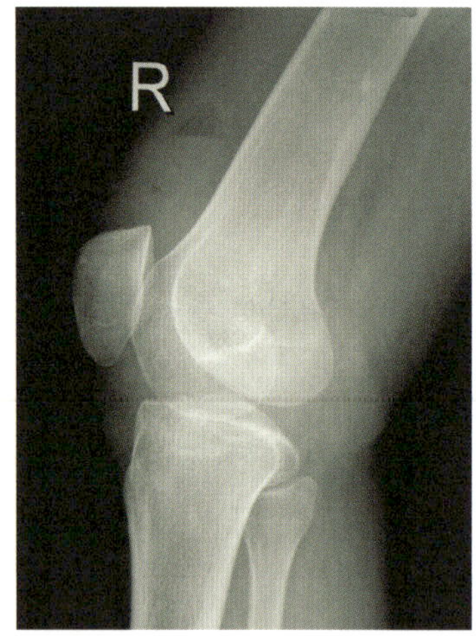

Patient	When will I receive the results?
Radiographer	You can discuss the results with your doctor during your upcoming appointment.
Patient	Thank you.
Radiographer	You're welcome, sir.

* examination table : 촬영 테이블, * under : 밑, 아래

B Reviewing Useful Expressions

1 I'll be exposed to radiation twice.

2 Don't worry, sir. The radiation dose is very low.

3 Your doctor needs the X-rays to diagnose any potential issues with your knee bones.

4 Please lie down on the examination table.

5 Please turn to your side.

6 Position one of your legs out in front of the other and slightly bend your knees.

7 You can discuss the results with your doctor during your upcoming appointment.

C Role playing

상황 ❶

방사선사 William Davis님

환자 저 여기 있습니다.

방사선사 환자분이 받으실 검사는 무릎 전면과 측면 촬영입니다.

환자 그 검사는 어떤 검사인가요?

방사선사 2장의 사진을 찍을 건데요, 전면과 측면 무릎 사진입니다. 따라서 환자분은 2번 X선 촬영을 하시게 될 겁니다.

환자 위험하지 않나요? 난 2번이나 X선을 받게 될 테니까요.

방사선사 걱정하지 마십시오. 환자분. 방사선의 양은 매우 적은 양입니다. 그리고 담당 의사선생님은 환자분의 무릎 뼈의 이상 유무를 찾으려고 X선 사진을 필요하다고 하십니다.

환자 아 그렇군요. 알겠습니다.

방사선사 환자분, 탈의실로 가셔서 옷을 벗고 병원 가운으로 갈아 입도록 하세요.

환자 바지도 벗어야 하나요?

방사선사 네, 환자분. 벗은 다음 병원 가운을 입으세요.

환자 알겠습니다.

상황 ❷

(촬영실에서 검사를 시행한다.)

방사선사 검사테이블에 누우십시오.

환자 여기요?

방사선사 네 환자분. 환자분 다리 아래 촬영판을 놓을테니 똑바로 누우십시오. 움직이지 마세요.

(방사선사가 X선을 조사한다.)

방사선사 환자분, 환자분의 측면으로 돌아서세요. 측면 사진을 찍겠습니다. 아래쪽 다리를 반대쪽 다리 앞으로 내밀어 약간 구부리세요.

환자 알겠습니다. 이렇게요?

방사선사 좋습니다. 그렇게요. 촬영하는 동안 움직이지 마세요.

환자 네 알겠습니다.

(방사선사가 X선을 조사한다.)

방사선사 검사가 끝났습니다. 일어나셔서 탈의실로 가서 옷을 갈아입으세요.

환자 언제 결과를 알 수 있나요.

방사선사 환자분이 진료를 예약한 날에 담당 의사선생님에게 결과를 문의하시면 됩니다.

환자 감사합니다.

방사선사 천만에요.

D Quiz

1 We'll ( ) two images, one from the front and one from the side.

2 Don't worry sir. The radiation dose is very ( ).

3 Lie down straight while I place the board ( ) your legs.

4 Please remain ( ) while I take the X-ray.

5 You can ( ) the results with your doctor during your upcoming appointment.

정답 take / low / under / still / discuss

E Translate Korean into English

1 2장의 사진을 찍을 건데요, 전면과 측면사진입니다.

2 방사선의 양은 무시할 정도로 적은 양입니다.

3 환자분, 환자분의 측면으로 돌아서세요. 측면 사진을 찍겠습니다.

4 아래쪽 다리를 반대쪽 다리 앞으로 내밀어 약간 구부리세요.

TIP! put

❶ **놓다** put this down there. (거기에 내려놓아라.) / stay put.(don't move.) / put it in. (안에 놓아라.) / put it out. (밖에~) / put it down. (아래에~) / put it up. (위에~)
❷ **변화시키다.** put Korean into English. (한국어를 영어로 번역하라.)
❸ **투자하다.** put your money into it. (돈 좀 투자해 봐요.)
❹ **값을 매기다.** I put our damage at ₩100,000. (손해를 100,000원으로 매겼다.)

Chapter 5

응급실에서 팔 검사하기

A Dialogue

SITUATION 1 I'll take care of the positioning and make you as comfortable as possible.

Nurse Good afternoon. We have a patient here from the Emergency Room for an X-ray of the right elbow, both front and side views. It's a trauma case, checking for any potential fractures.

Radiographer I understand.

Radiographer to the Nurse Could I please have the referral slip? The patient's name is Sophia Miller.

Nurse That's correct.

Radiographer Alright, let's bring the patient into the X-ray room.

Radiographer to the Nurse Could you take off the arm sling?

Nurse Of course.

Patient	Ouch... My arm hurts a lot!
Nurse to Patient	Ma'am, use your other hand to support your arm while I remove the sling.
Patient	Alright, please be gentle.
Radiographer to the Patient	Ma'am, have a seat in this chair facing the examination table. Can you try to move your arm?
Patient	No, moving it hurts.
Radiographer	What happened to your arm?
Patient	I was playing volleyball with my friends, and I tripped and fell.

* trauma : 외상, * sling : 붕대, * volleyball : 배구

SITUATION ❷

Radiographer	I'll position your arm on the examination table and place your elbow on the board. Please keep your arm still.
Patient	Sure.
Radiographer	I'll take care of the positioning and make you as comfortable as possible. Does it hurt when I position your arm like this?

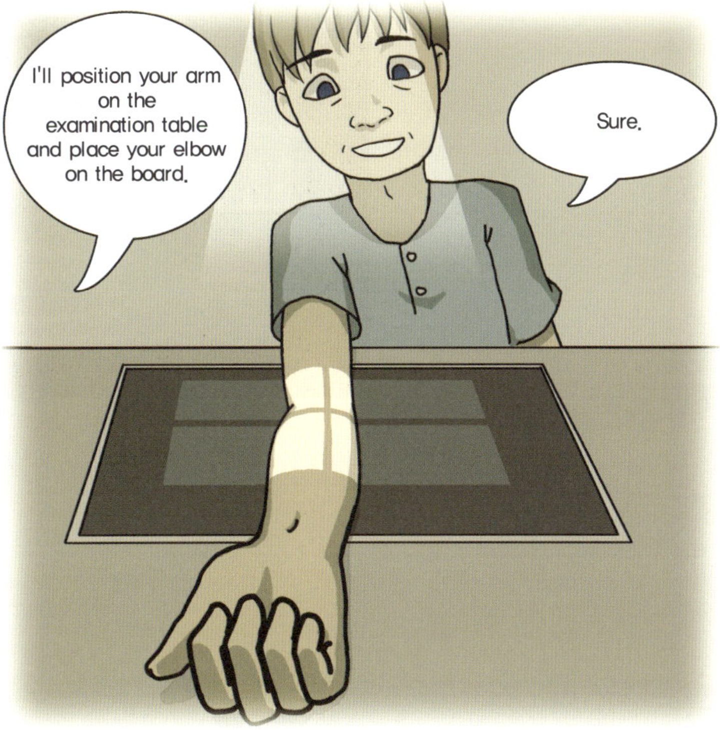

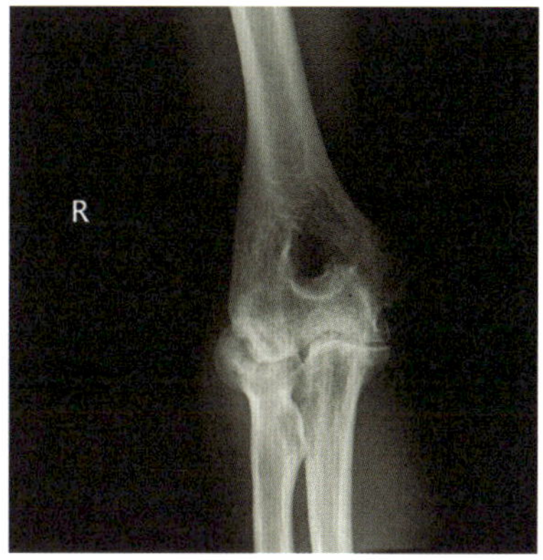

Patient No, just please don't stretch it. Even a slight movement hurts.

Radiographer Don't worry, I won't. Your elbow appears swollen. I'll focus on X-rays of that area. Please stay still.

Patient Are we done?

Radiographer Not yet, ma'am. That was just the front view. Now, I'll position your arm again to take a side view.

Patient Aahhh...

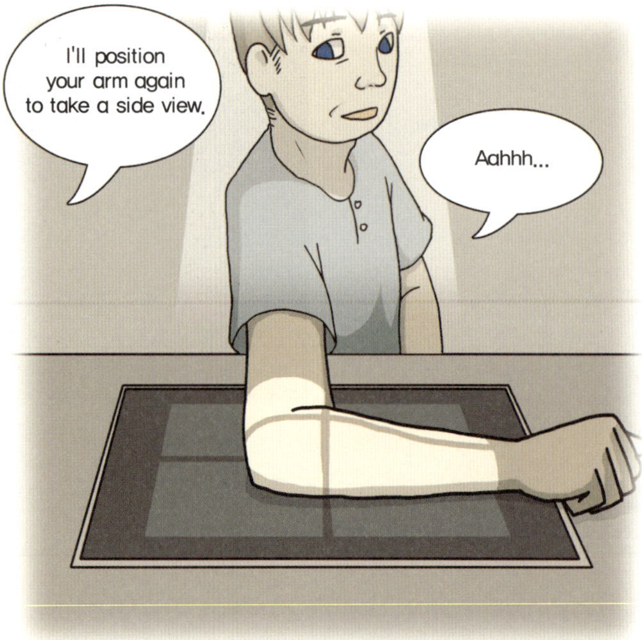

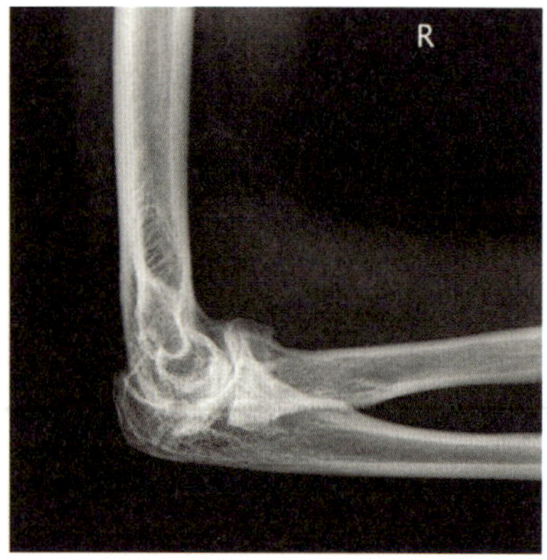

Radiographer Does moving your arm a bit cause any discomfort?

Patient No, but please avoid touching my elbow.

Radiographer No worries, I won't touch it. I'll gently rest it on the board. Alright, please stay still.

Radiographer The examination is complete. You'll be taken back to the emergency room.

Patient Okay, thank you.

Radiographer You're welcome.

* rest : ~에 두다. 얹다.

SITUATION ③

Radiographer Patient Sophia Miller?

Patient Yes, I'm here again.

Radiographer How are you feeling?

Patient I'm doing fine. I just can't play volleyball yet. They've put this cast on my elbow.

Radiographer Alright, ma'am. Let's proceed into the X-ray room.

Patient Okay.

Radiographer Ma'am, please have a seat in this chair facing the examination table, and I'll position your arm. Rest it here on the board.

Patient Alright.

Radiographer Please remain still. (click!)

Patient Is there an additional X-ray view required?

Radiographer Yes, ma'am, the side view. I'll adjust your arm like this. Okay, stay in that position. Please don't move. (click!)

Radiographer Ma'am, the exam is finished. You can get your results from your doctor.

Patient Okay, thank you.

Radiographer My pleasure.

B Reviewing Useful Expressions

1 We have a patient here from the Emergency Room for an X-ray.

2 Let's bring the patient into the X-ray room.

3 Have a seat in this chair facing the examination table.

4 Moving it hurts.

5 What happened to your arm?

6 I'll take care of the positioning and make you as comfortable as possible.

7 I'll position your arm again.

8 You'll be taken back to the emergency room.

C Role playing

상황 ❶

(외상으로 오른쪽 팔꿈치가 부운 20대 여성이 간호사와 함께 응급실에 들어온다.
환자는 팔에 삼각붕대를 멘 상태이다.)

간호사 안녕하세요. 응급실에서 오른쪽 팔꿈치 전면과 측면 사진이 필요한 환자를 모시고 왔습니다. 외상을 입은 것 같은데, 아마 골절인 것 같습니다.

방사선사 알겠습니다.

방사선사가 환자에게 안녕하세요. 검사 의뢰서를 주시겠어요? 환자 이름은 Sophia Miller이군요.

간호사 맞습니다.

방사선사 알겠습니다. 환자를 촬영실 안으로 옮기도록 합시다.

방사선사가 간호사에게 환자의 팔걸이 붕대를 제거해 주시겠어요?

간호사 네. 그렇게 하지요.

환자 아아... 팔이 정말 아파요.

간호사가 환자에게 제가 이 팔걸이 붕대를 제거하는 동안 반대 손으로 팔을 받쳐주세요.

환자 알겠습니다. 살살 해주세요.

방사선사가 환자에게 환자분, 검사테이블로 향한 상태로 이 의자에 앉아 주십시오.
팔을 움직일 수 있나요?

환자 아니요. 움직이면 아파요.

방사선사 어쩌다 팔을 다치셨나요?

환자 친구와 배구를 하다가 걸려 넘어졌어요.

상황 ❷

방사선사 환자분 팔을 촬영 테이블에, 그리고 다른 쪽 팔꿈치는 촬영판에 올려 놓겠습니다. 팔을 움직이지 마세요.

환자 알겠습니다.

방사선사 제가 자세를 잡을 터이니 환자분은 가능한 편한 자세를 유지하세요. 제가 환자분의 팔을 이렇게 자세를 취하면 아픈가요?

환자 아니요. 내 팔을 펴지만 말아 주세요. 조금만 움직여도 아파요.

방사선사　걱정 마세요. 그렇게 하지 않을께요. 팔꿈치가 부어 있군요. 그 부분을 중심으로 X선 촬영을 하겠습니다. 그 상태를 그대로 유지해 주세요.

(방사선사가 X선을 조사한다.)

환자　끝났나요?

방사선사　아직 끝나지 않았습니다. 지금은 정면 사진만 촬영했습니다. 이제 측면사진을 촬영하겠습니다. 다시 환자분 팔의 자세를 잡도록 하겠습니다.

환자　아아....

방사선사　제가 팔을 조금 움직였는데 아픕니까?

환자　아니요. 내 팔꿈치를 건드리지만 말아주세요.

방사선사　걱정마세요. 이제 팔을 촬영판에 올려놓겠습니다. 좋습니다. 그대로 계세요.

(방사선사가 X선을 조사한다.)

방사선사　검사가 끝났습니다. 환자분을 응급실도 보내드리겠습니다.

환자　네, 감사합니다.

방사선사　천만에요

상황 ❸

(2주후 환자가 팔에 깁스 한 상태로 외래를 통해 검사를 받으러 옴.)

방사선사　Sophia Miller님 계신가요?

환자　예 여기 다시 왔습니다.

방사선사　좀 어떠신가요?

환자 좋습니다. 아직 배구는 할 수 없어요. 의료진들이 팔에 깁스를 했어요.

방사선사 알겠습니다. 환자분. 촬영실 안으로 들어가시죠.

환자 알겠습니다.

방사선사 환자분 의자에 앉은 다음 검사테이블로 향해 주십시오. 팔의 자세를 잡도록 하겠습니다. 팔을 여기 촬영판 위에 올려놓으세요.

환자 알겠습니다.

방사선사 움직이지 마세요.

(방사선사가 X선을 조사한다. 찰칵!)

환자 촬영할 사진이 또 있나요?

방사선사 예 환자분, 측면 사진입니다. 환자분 팔을 이렇게 자세를 잡도록 하겠습니다. 좋습니다. 그런 식으로 자세를 유지하세요. 움직이지 마세요.

(방사선사가 X선을 조사한다. 찰칵!)

방사선사 환자분 검사가 끝났습니다. 검사 결과를 보시려면 담당 의사선생님께 가셔야 합니다.

환자 알겠습니다. 감사합니다.

방사선사 천만에요.

D Quiz

1 Have a seat in this chair ( ) the examination table.

2 Patient: Moving it hurts.

3 Radiographer: What (   ) to your arm?

4 I will (   ) your arm on the examination table and (   ) your elbow on the board.

5 I'll (   ) your arm again

정답 position / place / position / happened / facing

E Translate Korean into English

1 환자를 촬영실 안으로 옮기도록 합시다.

2 환자분, 검사테이블로 향한 상태로 이 의자에 앉아 주십시오.

3 제가 자세를 잡을 터이니 환자분은 가능한 편한 자세를 유지하세요.

4 지금은 정면 사진 만 촬영했습니다. 이제 측면사진을 촬영하겠습니다.

TIP! Do

❶ **~하다.** What can I do for you. (무엇을 도와드릴까요?) / I will move your arm, make yourself comfortable as possible.
❷ **종사하다.** I am an engineer. (제 직업은 엔지니어입니다.) / What do you do? (직업이 무엇입니까?)
❸ **영향을 주다.** The medicine will do you good. (그 약을 복용하면 좋아질 겁니다.)
❹ **의지의 강조** Do come again! (꼭 또 오십시오!)
❺ **좋다, 충분하다.** That will do. (그것으로 충분하다.)
❻ **관용구** I did the dish. (설거지를 했다.) / I'm doing my face. (화장을 하고 있다.) / I did my hair. (머리 손질을 했다.) / Job well done! (잘했어!)

Chapter 6

응급실에서 복부검사하기

A Dialogue

SITUATION 1 Is it alright if we move you a bit?

Nurse: Hello, we have a patient here from the ER who needs to be admitted. This is a case of a 40-year-old woman with abdominal pain, and we need a STAT plain abdominal X-ray.

Radiographer: Could I see the referral slip, please?

Nurse: Here it is

Radiographer: The patient's name is Emily Brown, correct?

Nurse: Yes, that's correct.

Radiographer: Alright, is it possible to move the patient onto the X-ray table?

Nurse: Yes, it's possible, but we'll need to assist her. Getting up is difficult for her due to the pain.

Radiographer to the Patient	Ma'am, we're going to transfer you to the X-ray table. Is it alright if we move you a bit?
Patient	Yes, that's fine.
Radiographer	You don't need to get up. We'll use the blanket you're lying on to carry you and move you.
Patient	Yes, I think I can manage that.
Radiographer to the Nurse	Okay, let's do it. One, two, three···

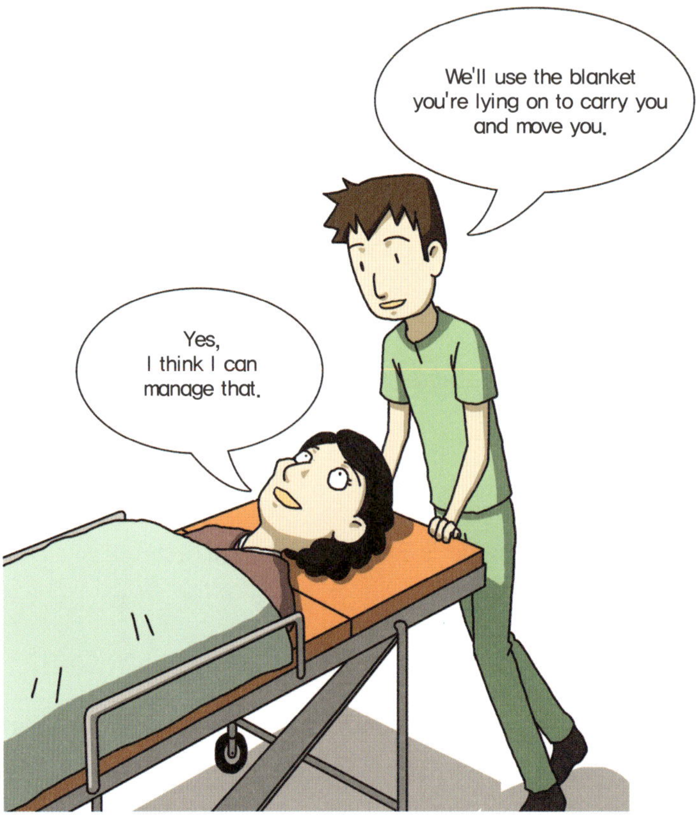

* STAT : Immediately, At Once 지금 당장, 즉시 - 어원 : statim(라틴) 즉시

SITUATION ❷

Radiographer to the Nurse	Please wear this lead gown for your protection while I take the X-ray.
Nurse	Thank you.
Radiographer to the Patient	Alright, ma'am, please stay still. Hold your breath... (click!)
Patient	Okay.
Patient	Ma'am, you can breathe comfortably now.
Nurse	Are we done?
Patient	Yes. Let's transfer the patient back to the stretcher.
Nurse	Okay, I'll take the patient to the surgical ward. What about the results? Can we get an initial reading?
Patient	Certainly. Our on-duty resident will provide you with an initial report. The official report will be forwarded to the ward. Alternatively, you can inquire with the receptionist on duty.
Nurse	Thank you.

* an initial reading 1차 판독, 정밀판독 전에 시행하는 간단한 판독

B Reviewing Useful Expressions

1 This is a case of a 40-year-old woman with abdominal pain, and we need a STAT plain abdominal X-ray.

2 Ma'am, we're going to transfer you to the X-ray table. Is it alright if we move you a bit?

3 We'll use the blanket you're lying on to carry and move you.

4 Let's transfer the patient back to the stretcher.

5 You can inquire with the receptionist on duty.

C Role playing

상황 1

(환자가 간호사와 함께 이동 테이블에 실려 들어온다.)

간호사 안녕하세요. 입원등록 절차를 위해 응급실에서 환자를 데려왔습니다.
이 환자는 복통을 호소하는 40세 여성의 환자로 응급 복부 촬영이 필요합니다.

방사선사 검사 의뢰서를 주시겠습니까?

간호사 네.

방사선사 환자의 이름은 Emily Brown이시군요.

간호사 맞습니다.

환자 네.

방사선사 좋습니다. 촬영테이블로 옮길 수 있을까요?

간호사 네, 가능은 한데요, 우리가 환자를 운반해서 이동해야 합니다. 환자가 일어나기 어렵습니다. 환가가 고통스러워해요.

방사선사가 환자에게 환자분, 우리가 환자분을 X선 테이블로 옮기려고 합니다. 환자분을 조금만 움직이려 하는데 괜찮으시겠어요?

환자 예, 물론이지요.

방사선사 환자분은 일어서면 안됩니다. 우리가 환자분이 누워있는 담요를 사용해서 옮기겠습니다.

환자 예, 저는 견딜 수 있을 것 같군요.

방사선사가 간호사에게 좋습니다. 자, 해봅시다.

(간호사와 함께 환자를 촬영대로 들어 옮긴다.)

하나, 둘, 셋...

상황 2

방사선사가 간호사에게 간호사분은 제가 촬영하는 동안 방사선을 막도록 이 납가운을 입도록 하세요.

간호사 감사합니다.

방사선사가 환자에게 좋습니다. 움직이지 마세요. 숨을 멈추고... 숨을 참고... 그대로 계세요.

환자 알겠습니다.

(방사선사가 X선을 조사한다. 찰칵!)

방사선사 환자분 이제 숨을 쉬어도 됩니다.

간호사 이제 마쳤나요?

방사선사 예, 스트레처에 환자를 옮기도록 합시다.

간호사 예, 제가 지금 외과병동으로 환자를 모시고 가겠습니다. 그런데 결과는 어떡하지요? 1차 판독을 받을 수 있나요?

방사선사 예. 당직의가 당신에게 1차 판독결과를 드릴 겁니다. 저희는 병동으로 정식 판독결과를 병동으로 보내드리겠습니다. 아니면 당직 접수 담당자에게 결과를 전화로 문의할 수 있습니다.

간호사 감사합니다.

D Quiz

1 ( ) up is difficult for her due to the pain.

2 Is it alright if we move you ( )?

3 We'll ( ) the blanket you're lying on to carry and move you.

4 ( ) this lead gown for your protection while I take the X-ray.

정답 wear / use / a bit / getting

E Translate Korean into English

1 우리가 환자분을 X선 테이블로 옮기려고 합니다.

2 환자분을 조금만 움직이려 하는데 괜찮으시겠어요?

3 환자분은 일어서면 안됩니다.

4 우리가 환자분이 누워있는 담요를 사용해서 옮기겠습니다.

5 환자분 이제 숨을 쉬어도 됩니다.

TIP! get

1. **구하다.** I want to get a computer.
2. **이해하다.** I don't get it. (난 이해가 안가.)
3. **~상태로 되다.** I'm getting excited! (난 흥분되었어!)
4. **병에 걸리다.** I got a cold. (난 감기에 걸렸어.)
5. **~하도록 하다.** I'll get a doctor to help me.
6. **가져다주다.** Get me that book. (저 책 좀 가져다 줘.)
7. **관용구** get up (일어나다.) / get on (올라타다.) / get to (~에 이르다.)

Chapter 7

조영제를 사용한 방사선 검사하기

A Dialogue

SITUATION ❶ Have you received a similar injection before?

Radiographer Are you Ms. Grace Wilson?

Patient Yes, that's me.

Radiographer (for a female patient) Are you married? Do you think you could be pregnant?

Patient I'm single. No, I'm not pregnant.

Radiographer Have you ever had this kind of examination before?

Patient No, this is my first time.

Radiographer Please read and sign the consent form.

Patient Okay.

Radiographer Do you have any food or medicine allergies?

Patient No, I don't have any allergies to food or medicine.

Radiographer Please proceed to the dressing room and remove all metal objects from your body.

(During the examination)

Radiographer Please lie down on the examination table and remain still.

Patient Sure.

Radiographer Ma'am, hold your breath for me. (click!) You may now breathe and relax.

SITUATION ❷

Radiographer Please stretch out your hand. I'll be using a butterfly needle for the contrast injection. First, I'll administer a test dose before the full one. Have you received a similar injection before?

Patient No.

Radiographer If you start feeling sick or experience any abnormal sensations, please let me know immediately.

Patient Sure, I will.

Radiographer Do you notice any unusual sensations, ma'am?

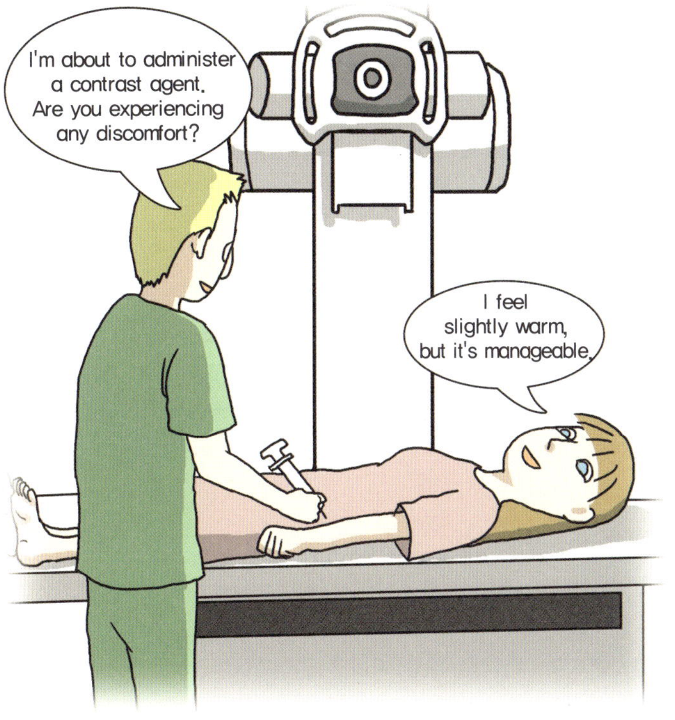

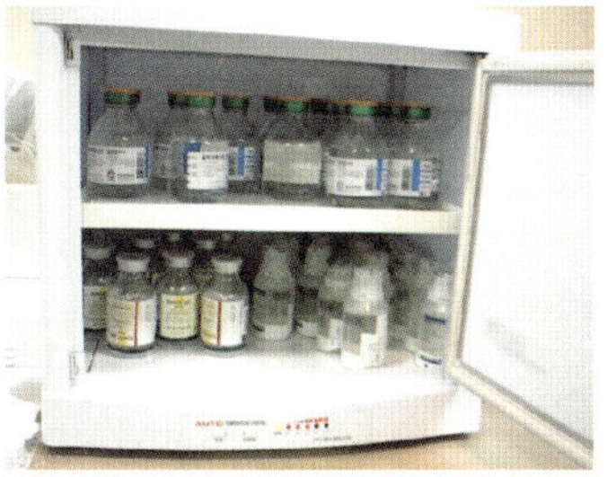

[조영제의 보관]

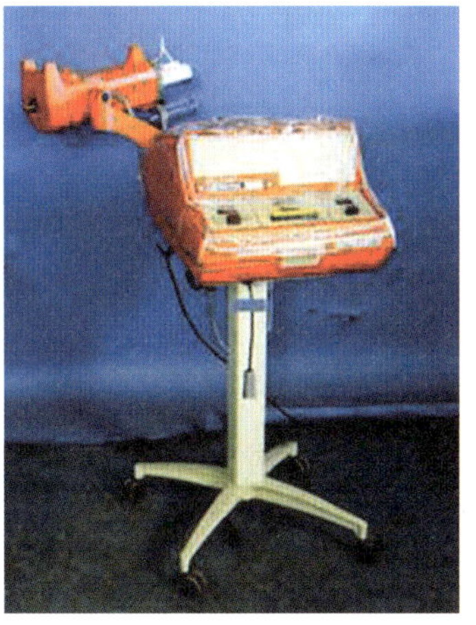

Patient	No, I feel fine.
Radiographer	I'm about to administer a contrast agent. Are you experiencing any discomfort?
Patient	I feel slightly warm, but it's manageable.
Radiographer	Don't worry if you feel warm; it's normal.
Patient	Okay.
Radiographer	Please don't hesitate to let me know if you experience itchiness, difficulties with breathing or swallowing, dizziness, or any other unusual symptoms. I'll be here to assist you.

Patient Thank you, that's very kind of you.

(After the examination)

Radiographer The examination is finished. You can follow up with your doctor regarding your test results.

Patient Alright.

Radiographer Make sure to drink plenty of water. It will help flush out the contrast agent from your system.

Patient Thank you, I appreciate it.

* test dose : 시험용 분량, * full dose : 주사액 전량, * itchiness : 가려운 ; 좀이 쑤시는, swallowing : 삼키기, dizziness : 어지러움, * system : 인체, 인체의 기관, * consent form : 검사 동의서

B Reviewing Useful Expressions

1 Are you married? Do you think you could be pregnant?

2 Have you ever had this kind of examination before?

3 Please read and sign the consent form.

4 Do you have any food or medicine allergies?

5 Please stretch out your hand.

6 I'll be using a butterfly needle for the contrast injection.

7 I'll administer a test dose before the full one.

8 If you start feeling sick or experience any abnormal sensations, please let me know immediately.

9 Do you notice any unusual sensations?

10 Make sure to drink plenty of water. It will help flush out the contrast agent from your system.

C Role playing

상황 1

(검사 전 방사선사가 환자에게 검사에 대한 내용을 설명한다.)

방사선사 환자분이 Grace Wilson이신가요?

환자 예, 제가 맞습니다.

방사선사 (여성 환자에게) 결혼하셨나요? 임신 가능성이 있으신가요?

환자 미혼입니다. 임신 중이 아닙니다.

방사선사 이전에 이와 같은 검사를 받으신 적이 있나요?

환자 아니요. 이번이 처음입니다.

방사선사 책상 위에 있는 검사 동의서를 작성해 주세요.

환자 알겠습니다.

방사선사 환자분은 음식이나 약제에 대해 알러지를 가지고 있나요?

환자 아니요. 저는 음식이나 약물에 대해 알러지가 없습니다.

방사선사 탈의실에 가셔서 가지고 계신 모든 금속 물질을 제거해 주십시오.

(검사가 진행된다.)

방사선사 검사테이블에 누워주십시오. 움직이지 마세요.

환자 알겠습니다.

방사선사 환자분 숨을 멈춰주세요. (찰칵!) 이제 숨을 쉬고 편하게 계세요.

상황 ❷

방사선사 손을 저에게 내밀어 보세요. 조영제 투여를 위해 나비 바늘을 이용하겠습니다. 주사약 전량을 주입하기 전에 우선 시험용 분량을 투여 하겠습니다. 이전에 이와 유사한 주사약을 맞은 적이 있나요?

환자 아니오.

방사선사 만일 환자분의 기분이 불쾌하게 느껴지거나 이상한 느낌이 들면 즉시 저에게 알려주세요.

환자 예 알겠습니다.

방사선사 환자분 이상한 느낌이 드시나요?

환자 아니요. 괜찮아요.

방사선사 이제 조영제를 주사하고 있습니다. 어떤 불편함이라도 느끼시나요?

환자 조금 따뜻한 느낌이 들지만 견딜 만합니다.

방사선사 환자분이 따뜻한 느낌이 있다면, 걱정 마세요. 그건 정상입니다.

방사선사 만일 환자분이 느끼시기에 가려움증, 호흡이나 삼키기가 곤란하시거나, 현기증 혹은 이상한 증상이 있으시면 즉시 제게 알려주십시오. 제가 환자분을 보살피기 위해 여기에 있겠습니다.

환자 　알겠습니다. 고맙습니다. 정말 친절한 분이시군요.

(검사 후)

방사선사 　검사가 끝났습니다. 환자분은 약속하신 날에 담당 의사선생님을 찾아가시면 됩니다. 그 분이 환자분의 검사 결과를 설명해 드릴 겁니다.

환자 　알겠습니다.

방사선사 　환자분은 물을 많이 드셔야 합니다. 환자분 몸으로부터 조영제를 제거 하는데 도움이 될 것입니다.

환자 　알겠습니다. 감사합니다.

D Quiz

1 Have you ( ) had this kind of examination before?

2 Please read and sign the ( ).

3 Please ( ) your hand.

4 I'll be here to ( ) you.

5 Make sure to drink ( ) of water. It will help ( ) the contrast agent from your system.

정답 flush out / plenty / assist / stretch out / consent form / ever

E Translate Korean into English

1 결혼하셨나요? 임신 가능성이 있으신가요?

2 책상 위에 있는 검사 동의서를 작성해 주세요.

3 환자분은 음식이나 약제에 대해 알레르기를 가지고 있나요? 혹시 있다면? 무엇인가요?

4 만일 환자분의 기분이 불쾌하게 느껴지거나 이상한 느낌이 들면 즉시 저에게 알려주세요.

TIP! take

① **앗아가다.** You take my pencil. (네가 내 연필을 가져갔다.)
② **가져가다.** Take this! (이것을 가져가시오!)
③ **받아들이다.** Do you take me a fool? (나를 바보로 생각하니?)
④ **받다.** I took a medical advice. (나는 의사의 진단을 받았다.)
⑤ **걸리다.** It takes days. (며칠 걸린다.)
⑥ **취하다.** Take a deep breath. (숨을 깊이 들이 쉬세요.)

Chapter 8

CT 검사하기

A Dialogue

SITUATION 1 Your examination will involve the injection of a contrast agent.

Patient	Good afternoon. I'd like to schedule a CT scan for my head.
Radiographer	Good afternoon, Sir. May I have your name, please?
Patient	James Moor.
Radiographer	Your request is for a Cranial CT scan with contrast.
Patient	That's correct.
Radiographer	Let me check our schedule, sir. We have an available slot tomorrow at 9 a.m. Does that work for you?
Patient	Ah, yes, I'll take that.

Radiographer	We have some preparation instructions for this examination. Please follow what's written on this appointment slip.
Patient	Okay.
Radiographer	Sir, during the evening before your scan, have a regular meal. After midnight you need to fast from food and drinks except for medications if you're on any.
Patient	Got it.
Radiographer	Then return here about 5 minutes before your scheduled time.
Patient	Sure.
Radiographer	Please bring this appointment slip, ultrasound, X-ray, or old CT scan results if you have any from other hospitals. Also, don't forget to bring your serum creatinine results.
Patient	Why do I need that?
Radiographer	Because your examination involves an injection of a contrast agent.
Patient	Okay, thank you. See you tomorrow then.

SITUATION ❷

Radiographer	Did you follow the instructions given to you?
Patient	Of course.
Radiographer	Sir, may I have your serum creatinine results? Do you have any test results from another hospital?
Patient	Here they are.
Radiographer	Let me check your serum creatinine first... okay, it's normal. Do you have any allergies to food or medications?
Patient	No.
Radiographer	Okay, sir, please fill out this information sheet, then read and sign the consent form.
Patient	I'm done. What do I do now?
Radiographer	Let's go inside the scanning room.
Patient	Okay.
Radiographer	Please lie down straight on the examination table.
Patient	Can I have that blanket? This room is cold.
Radiographer	Yes, sir. Please lie down, and I'll put the blanket on you.
Patient	Thanks.

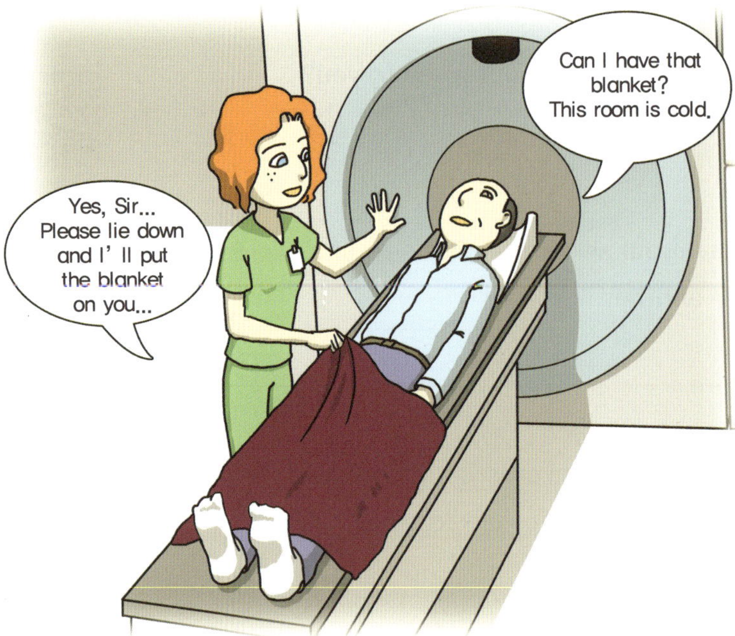

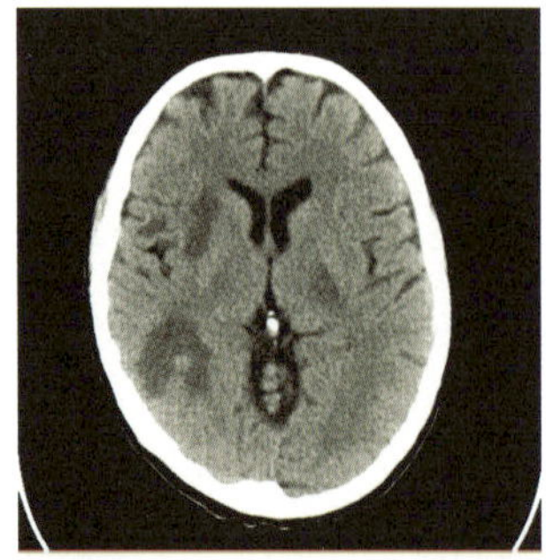

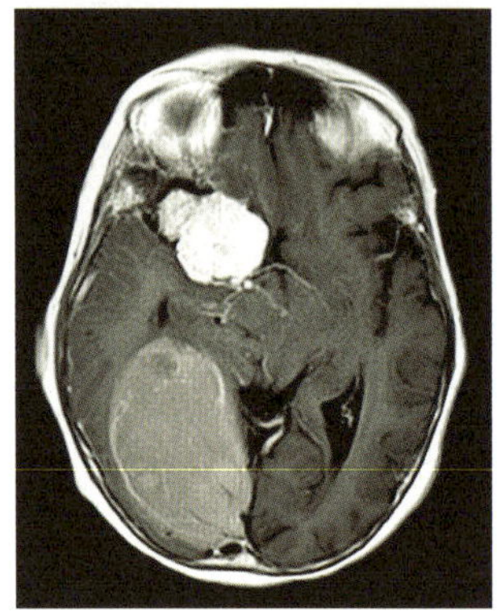

Radiographer I will do the initial scanning. Please be still.

Patient Okay.

Radiographer Sir, the doctor will now insert a butterfly needle in your arm and will do the test dose of the contrast agent.

SITUATION ❸

Patient Good morning, Doctor.

Doctor I'm the resident-on-duty here. Can I have your arm, please? I will insert this butterfly needle. It might sting a bit, but it's manageable. Please inform us immediately if you feel unwell or experience any abnormal sensations, like difficulty in breathing and swallowing, itchiness, or discomfort. We need to monitor for signs of allergies.

Patient Sure, Doctor.

Doctor How are you feeling, sir? Do you notice anything unusual?

Patient Nothing unusual. I feel fine.

Doctor I'm now administering the full dose. Do you feel any discomfort?

Patient No.

Doctor Full dose administered. Please don't hesitate to inform us if you experience any abnormal symptoms. We still need to watch for signs of allergies during this scan.

Patient Sure.

Radiographer We're ready to begin the scan, sir. Please try to remain still. The scan won't take too long.

(After the examination)

Radiographer Sir, the examination is finished. Allow me to assist you in getting up. Do you notice any abnormalities or discomfort?

Patient Not that I can tell. I feel fine.

Radiographer I'll now remove the butterfly needle from your arm.

Patient I'm hungry. Can I eat now?

Radiographer	Yes, sir.
Patient	So, when can I get the results?
Radiographer	You can follow up with your doctor. He will explain the results to you.
Patient	Thanks.
Radiographer	You're welcome, sir.

B Reviewing Useful Expressions

1 Your request is for a Cranial CT scan with contrast.

2 Let me check our schedule. Sir, we have an available slot tomorrow at 9 a.m.

3 Sir, during the evening before your scan, have a regular meal. After midnight you need to fast from food and drinks.

4 You need to fast from food and drinks except for medications if you're on any.

5 Then return here about 5 minutes before your scheduled time.

6 Please bring this appointment slip, ultrasound, X-ray, or old CT scan results if you have any from other hospitals.

7 Did you follow the instructions given to you?

8 Please fill out this information sheet, then read and sign the consent form.

9 Please lie down, and I'll put the blanket on you.

10 Sir, the doctor will now insert a butterfly needle in your arm and will do the test dose of the contrast agent.

11 We're ready to begin the scan, sir. Please try to remain still. The scan won't take too long.

C Role playing

상황 ❶

환자	안녕하세요. 머리 CT 검사를 예약하러 왔습니다.
방사선사	안녕하세요. 환자분. 성함을 알려주세요.
환자	James Moor입니다.
방사선사	환자분 검사의뢰서에 따르면 조영제를 사용한 두개부 CT검사이군요.
환자	예 맞습니다.
방사선사	스케줄을 알아보겠습니다. 환자분 내일 아침 9시에 검사가 가능하겠네요. 그 시간이면 괜찮으신가요?
환자	아, 예... 그렇게 하겠습니다.
방사선사	검사를 하려면 준비 사항이 있습니다. 이 예약지에 나와 있는 지시사항을 따라주십시오.
환자	알겠습니다.
방사선사	환자분, 평소대로 저녁식사를 하신 다음 자정 이후로는 아무것도 먹거나 마시면 안 됩니다. 환자분이 평소에 드시는 약이 있다면 그 약 이외에는 금식 하셔야 합니다.
환자	예. 알겠습니다.

방사선사　그럼 예약 시간 5분전에 이곳으로 와주십시오.

환자　그렇게 하겠습니다.

방사선사　이 예약지와 만일 다른 병원에서 이와 같은 검사를 하셨다면 초음파, X선, 과거 CT 스캔 결과를 가져오세요. 그리고 혈청 크리아틴 검사결과를 가져오시는 것을 잊지 마세요.

환자　그것이 왜 필요한가요?

방사선사　왜냐하면 환자분 검사에는 조영제 투여가 포함되어 있기 때문입니다.

환자　알겠습니다. 그럼 내일 봅시다.

상황 ❷

(다음날)

방사선사　환자분에게 드린 지시사항 대로 하셨나요?

환자　물론이지요.

방사선사　환자분의 혈청 크리아틴을 주시겠어요? 다른 병원에서 나온 검사 결과를 가져오셨나요?

환자　여기 있습니다.

방사선사　우선 혈청 크리아틴을 확인하겠습니다. 좋습니다. 정상입니다. 환자분은 음식이나 어떤 약품에 대해 알레르기가 있나요?

환자　아니오.

방사선사　네, 환자분, 이 안내용지의 내용을 적어 주십시오. 그리고 나서 검사동의서를 읽으신 후에 사인해 주십시오.

환자　이 서류 작성을 다 마쳤습니다. 이제 무엇을 할까요?

방사선사　촬영실 안으로 들어가시지요.

환자 예.

(환자와 함께 촬영실 안으로 들어간다.)

방사선사 검사테이블에 똑바로 누어 주세요.

환자 담요 좀 덮어주세요. 방이 춥네요.

방사선사 예. 누워계십시요. 담요를 덮어 드리겠습니다.

환자 감사합니다.

방사선사 먼저 단순 촬영을 하겠습니다. 그대로 계세요.

환자 알겠습니다.

방사선사 환자분, 이제 환자분 팔에 나비주사를 넣고 조영제 주사약의 시험용 분량을 투여 하겠습니다.

(조영제 주사약의 실험용 분량을 투여 함)

상황 ❸

의사 안녕하세요. 환자분. 저는 의사 김이라고 합니다.

환자 안녕하세요. 의사선생님.

의사 저는 이곳 담당 전공의입니다. 환자분 팔을 보여주실까요? 제가 나비주사침을 놓겠습니다. 주사가 약간 아프지만 견딜만하실 겁니다. 만일 좋지 않은 느낌이나 호흡곤란, 삼키는데 있어서 어려움, 가려움증, 혹은 기타 불편한 증상 등등의 복부상 이상이 나타나면 즉시 우리에게 알려주세요. 우리는 알레르기 반응을 관찰해야 합니다.

환자 잘 알겠습니다.

(조영제 반응검사를 마친다.)

의사 환자분 기분이 좀 어떠십니까? 어떤 이상 증상이라도 느끼십니까?

환자 아무런 이상 증상이 없습니다. 기분이 좋습니다.

의사 이제 제가 전량을 주사하겠습니다. 어떤 불편한 점이라도 느껴집니까?

환자 아니요.

의사 모두 주사했습니다. 환자분, 만일 어떠한 이상한 점이나 혹은 복부에 이상한 증세가 느껴지면 즉시 우리에게 알려주세요. 우리는 계속 스캔이 진행되는 동안 알레르기 반응을 계속 관찰해야 합니다.

환자 예 알겠습니다.

방사선사 우리는 지금 촬영을 하고 있습니다. 환자분 움직이지 마세요. 촬영은 오래 걸리지 않을 겁니다.

(검사를 모두 마친다.)

방사선사 환자분 검사가 끝났습니다. 일어나도록 도와드리겠습니다. 환자분이 느끼시기에 어떤 이상한 증세라도 있나요?

환자 없습니다. 괜찮아요.

방사선사 이제 제가 나비 주사침을 제거하겠습니다.

환자 아, 예.. 좀 시장하군요. 지금 식사해도 되나요?

방사선사 예.

환자 그럼 언제 결과를 볼 수 있나요?

방사선사 진료예약 날짜에 담당의사 선생님을 만나시면 결과를 설명해 주실 겁니다.

환자 감사합니다.

방사선사 천만에요.

D Quiz

1 We have some ( ) for this examination. Please follow what's written on this appointment slip.

2 Did you follow the instructions ( ) to you?

3 Sir, we have an ( ) tomorrow at 9 am. Does that work for you?

4 You need to fast from food and drinks ( ) for medications if you're on any.

5 How are you feeling, sir? Do you notice anything ( )?

정답 unusual / except / available slot / given / preparation instructions

E Translate Korean into English

1 환자분 검사의뢰서에 따르면 조영제를 사용한 두개부 CT검사이군요.

2 검사를 하려면 준비 사항이 있습니다. 이 예약지에 나와 있는 지시사항을 따라주십시오.

3 환자분 움직이지 마세요. 촬영은 오래 걸리지 않을 겁니다.

4 환자분이 느끼시기에 어떤 이상한 증세라도 있나요?

5 이제 제가 나비 주사침을 제거하겠습니다.

TIP! **give**

- **주다.** He gave me a book.
- **안부를 보내다.** I will give you some instructions for you to follow.
- **(손을) 내밀다.** Please give me your hand.
- **~을 하다** 상용구 give a push (누르다.) / give up (포기하다.) / give in (속아 넘어가다.) / give away (줘버리다.) / give over (넘겨주다.)

Chapter 9

MRI 검사하기

A Dialogue

SITUATION ❶ Do you have any dental implants, a cardiac pacemaker, or any devices inside your body?

Radiographer	MRI Imaging Center. How can I assist you today?
Patient	My name is David Taylor, and I have an MRI exam scheduled for Monday at 9 a.m. Unfortunately, I won't be able to make it on that day. Is it possible to reschedule it for Tuesday at 1 p.m.?
Radiographer	Let me check for availability on Tuesday. Unfortunately, we don't have any openings until 4:00 p.m., unless there's a cancellation.
Patient	How about any time after 4 p.m.?
Radiographer	Great, we have 4:30 available. Is that time slot suitable for you?
Patient	Yes, that works for me.

Radiographer Let me confirm that. Your new appointment will be on Tuesday, October 10, at 4:30.

Patient Perfect. Thank you so much.

Radiographer You're welcome.

* Let me double check. 다시 한번 확인할게요.

SITUATION ❷

Radiographer Are you Mr. David Taylor?

Patient Yes.

Radiographer Are you here for an examination?

Patient Yes, I am. Here's my referral slip.

Radiographer Have you ever had surgery before?

Patient No, never.

Radiographer Do you have any dental implants, a cardiac pacemaker, or any devices inside your body?

Patient No, I don't have any of those.

Radiographer Do you have any heart conditions?

Patient No, my heart is healthy.

Radiographer Please go to the dressing room, change into the hospital gown, and remove all metals from your body.

Patient Okay.

Radiographer You will hear a lot of noise during the examination. Here are some earplugs for you to wear.

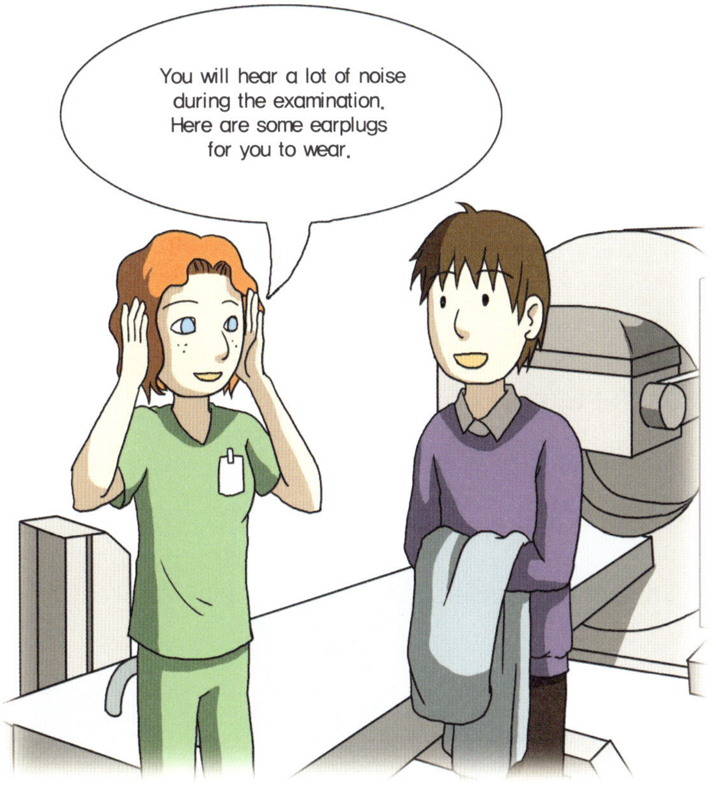

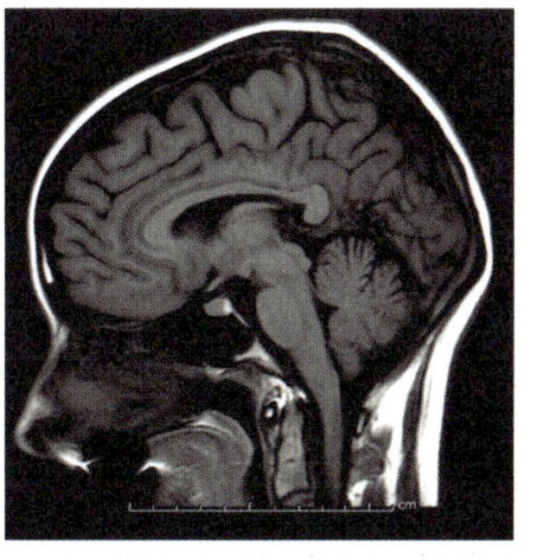

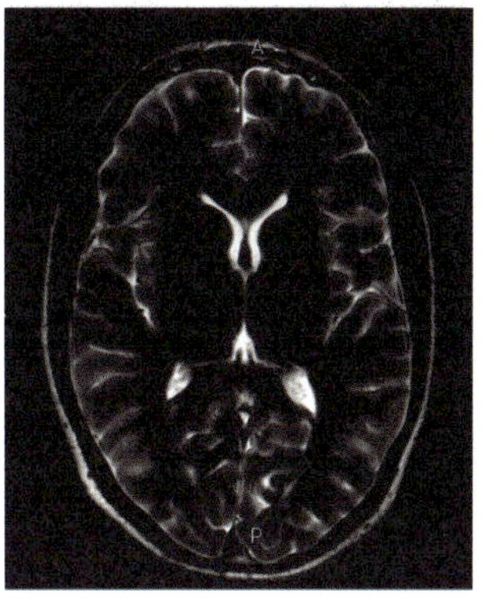

Patient　Certainly.

Radiographer　Please lie down on the examination table.

Patient　Right here? Okay.

(Examination)

Radiographer　Please remain still.

Radiographer　The examination is finished.

Radiographer　You can follow up with your doctor for the official results.

Patient　Alright, thank you very much.

* implants : 임플란트, 이식조직, * pacemaker : 심박동조절장치, * devices : 이식된 장치나 물건,
* metal objects : 금속물질, * earplug : 귀마개

B Reviewing Useful Expressions

1 Have you ever had surgery before?

2 Do you have any dental implants, a cardiac pacemaker, or any devices inside your body?

3 Remove all metals from your body.

4 You will hear a lot of noise during the examination.

5 Here are some earplugs for you to wear.

C Role playing

상황 1 전화로 예약을 변경하기

방사선사 MRI 검사실입니다. 무엇을 도와드릴까요?

환자 제 이름은 David Taylor입니다. 제가 월요일 오전9시에 MRI 검사가 예약이 되어 있어요. 그런데 그 날에 MRI 검사를 할 수 없네요. 가능하다면 화요일 오후 1시로 스케줄을 다시 잡아주실 수 있나요?

방사선사 그날 가능한 시간이 있는 지 체크해 보겠습니다.
(잠시 후)
만일 취소되는 환자가 없다면 오후 4시까지는 가능한 스케줄이 없네요.

환자 오후 4시 이후라면 어떤가요?

방사선사 좋습니다. 4시 30분에는 가능합니다. 그 시간으로 정하시겠습니까?

환자 예, 그 시간으로 하겠습니다.

방사선사 다시 한번 확인하겠습니다. 환자분의 새로운 예약은 10월 10일 화요일 오후 4시 30분입니다.

환자 맞아요. 정말 고맙습니다.

방사선사 천만에요.

상황 2

(검사 시행 전)

방사선사 환자분이 David Taylor씨 인가요?

환자 그렇습니다.

방사선사 환자분이 검사받으러 오셨나요?

환자　　예. 여기 검사의뢰서가 있습니다.

방사선사　　이전에 수술을 받으신 적이 있나요?

환자　　아니오.

방사선사　　환자분의 몸에 임플란트나 심박조절장치 혹은 이식된 장치가 있나요?

환자　　아니오. 저는 그런 것 없습니다.

방사선사　　심장질환이 있으십니까?

환자　　아니오. 제가 알기로는 제 심장은 괜찮습니다.

방사선사　　탈의실에 가셔서 검사용 가운으로 갈아입으시고, 가지고 계신 모든 금속 물질을 제거해 주세요.

환자　　예 알겠습니다.

방사선사　　검사하는 동안 기계에서 많은 소음이 날 겁니다. 소음 때문에 불편하실 수 있으니 귀마개를 착용해 주세요.

환자　　알겠습니다.

방사선사　　검사 테이블에 누우십시오.

환자　　여기요? 알겠습니다.

(검사 시행 중)

방사선사　　움직이지 마세요.

(검사 시행 후)

방사선사　　검사가 끝났습니다. 정식 검사결과를 보시려면 다시 담당 의사선생님을 찾아가십시오.

환자 : 예. 감사합니다.

D Quiz

1 Let me (   ) that. Your new appointment will be on Tuesday, October 10th, at 4:30.

2 (   ) you ever had surgery before?

3 Here are some (   ) for you to wear.

정답 earplugs / have / confirm

E Translate Korean into English

1 그 날 가능한 스케줄이 있는지 체크해 보겠습니다.

2 환자분의 몸에 임플란트나 심박조절장치 혹은 이식된 장치가 있나요?

3 가지고 계신 모든 금속 물질을 제거해 주세요.

4 검사하는 동안 기계에서 많은 소음이 날 겁니다.

5 소음 때문에 불편하실 수 있으니 귀마개를 착용해 주세요.

Chapter 10

위장 검사하기

A Dialogue

SITUATION 1 It will cause your stomach to expand for the examination.

Radiographer Have you eaten breakfast?

Patient No, I haven't. I'm quite hungry now.

Radiographer Do you have a necklace or a bra on?

Patient Yes, should I remove them?

Radiographer Ma'am, please go to the dressing room, take off your bra, change into the hospital gown, and remove your necklace and all metals from your body.

(Examination...)

Radiographer This is an effervescent agent. It will cause your stomach to expand for the examination. Please take the entire packet.

Patient Okay.

Radiographer Now, please drink some water. Just swallow it, no need to gargle. Afterwards, remove your shoes and get onto the examination table.

Patient Okay.

Radiographer Hold the cup with your left hand and follow the doctor's instructions.

Patient Alright, I understand.

Radiographer Follow the doctor’s instructions when the doctor asks you to hold the barium in your mouth, then only swallow it when the doctor directs to you.

Patient Okay.

Radiographer Once you've finished the contents of this cup, please place it on the rack.

Patient Okay.

Radiographer Now, turn onto your left side, lift your chin up, and listen to the doctor's instructions.

(After the examination)

Radiographer The examination is over.

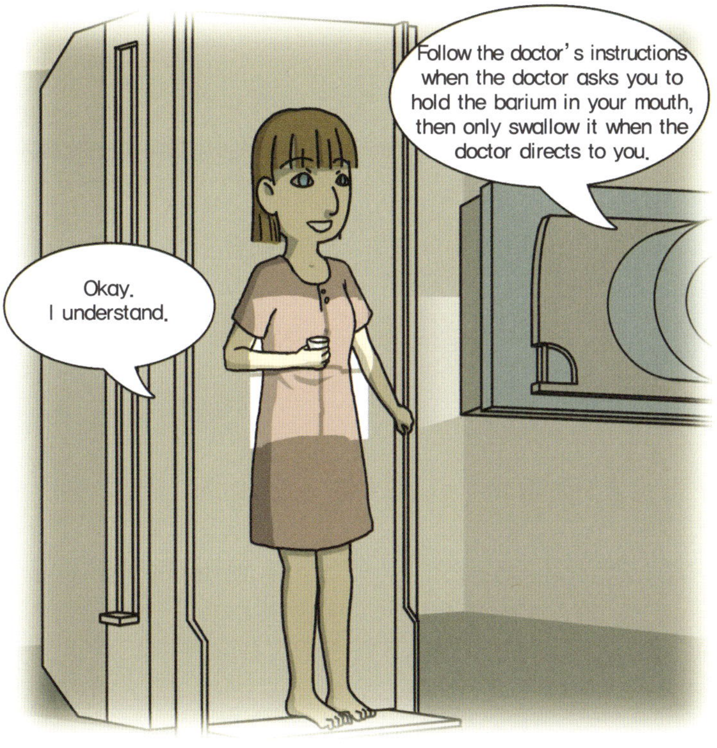

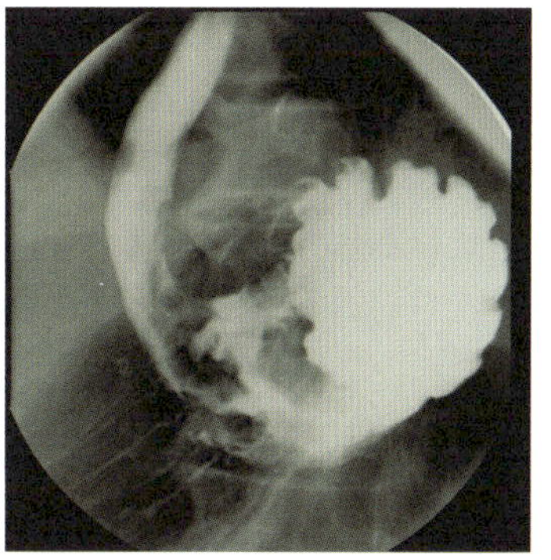

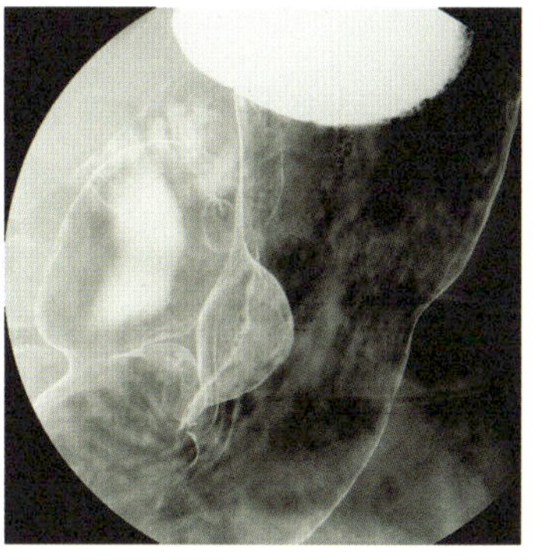

Patient	Can I eat now? I'm quite hungry.
Radiographer	Yes, you can eat now. Be sure to drink plenty of water, and you can discuss your results with your doctor.
Patient	Okay, thank you!

* robe : 긴 가운, * an effervescent agent : 가스를 발생시켜 위장을 부풀어 오르게 하기 위해 복용하는 전처치약, * Barium : 위장검사용 조영제, * swallow : 꿀꺽 삼키다., * cup rack : 컵 보관대

B Reviewing Useful Expressions

1 Please go to the dressing room, take off your bra, and change into the hospital gown.

2 Remove your necklace and all metals from your body.

3 It will cause your stomach to expand for the examination.

4 Please take the entire packet.

5 Please drink some water. Just swallow it, no need to gargle.

6 Turn onto your left side, lift your chin up, and listen to the doctor's instructions.

C Role playing

(검사 전 준비 상황)

방사선사 아침을 드셨나요?

환자 아니오. 아무것도 먹지 않았는데요, 지금 너무 배가 고파요.

방사선사 목걸이나 브라를 착용하고 계신가요?

환자 네, 다 제거해야 하나요?

방사선사 환자분, 탈의실로 가셔서 브라를 벗으시고 검사가운으로 갈아 입으세요. 그리고 목걸이와 몸에 있는 모든 금속 물질은 제거해 주세요.

(검사 중)

방사선사 이것은 가스를 발생시키는 약입니다. 이 약은 검사를 위해 환자분 위장을 부풀어 오르게 할 것입니다. 이 약을 전부 드세요.

환자 알겠습니다.

방사선사 물은 조금만 드세요. 가글은 하지 마시고 곧장 물을 삼키세요.
그리고 신발을 벗으시고 검사테이블로 올라오세요.

환자 예.

방사선사 왼손으로 컵을 잡으시고, 의사의 지시대로 따라주십시오.

환자 알겠습니다.

방사선사 의사가 환자분에게 바륨을 입에 물고 있으라고 하면, 지시대로 하세요.
그리고 의사가 바리움을 삼키라고 하면, 지시대로 하세요.

환자 네, 알겠습니다.

방사선사 환자분이 이 컵에 있는 것을 드신 후에는 컵 받침대에 놓아 주세요.

환자 알겠습니다.

방사선사 환자분 왼쪽으로 돌아주세요, 턱을 들어보세요, 그리고 의사의 지시를 잘 들어주세요.

(검사 시행 후)

환자 이제 식사를 해도 되나요? 배가 너무 고프네요.

방사선사 검사가 끝났습니다. 환자분은 이제 식사를 하실 수 있습니다. 그리고 물을 많이 드시고, 결과를 보시려면 진료예약 날짜에 담당의사 선생님께 가시면 됩니다.

환자 알겠습니다. 감사합니다.

D Quiz

1 Please go to the dressing room, (   ) your bra, and change into the hospital gown.

2 It will cause your stomach to (   ) for the examination.

3 Please drink some water. Just (   ) it, no need to gargle.

4 Afterwards, (   ) your shoes and get (   ) the examination table.

5 (   ) onto your left side, lift your chin up, and listen to the doctor's instructions.

정답 turn / onto / remove / swallow / expand / take off

E Translate Korean into English

1 목걸이와 몸에 있는 모든 금속 물질을 제거해 주세요.

2 이것은 가스를 발생시키는 약입니다. 이 약을 전부 드세요.

3 물은 조금만 드세요. 가글은 하지 마시고 곧장 물을 삼키세요.

4 의사가 바륨을 삼키라고 하면, 지시대로 하세요.

Chapter 11

대장 검사하기

A Dialogue

SITUATION ❶ Now please relax, we're going to insert this tube.

Radiographer	Have you had breakfast?
Patient	No, I was told not to eat.
Radiographer	Please proceed to the dressing room, take off your pants, change into the hospital gown, and remember to remove all accessories and any metals from your body.
Patient	Alright.
Radiographer	Did you follow the provided instructions?
Patient	Yes, I did.
Radiographer	Have you ever had your appendix removed?
Patient	No, I haven't.

Radiographer Great, please remove your shoes and get onto the examination table. Turn onto your left side.

Patient Okay.

Radiographer Now, relax your anal muscles. We're going to insert a tube into your anus. This might feel uncomfortable, but it won't hurt.

Patient Alright, I'm relaxed.

Radiographer I'm now going to pump barium through the inserted tube. Tighten your anal muscles so the Barium doesn't leak.

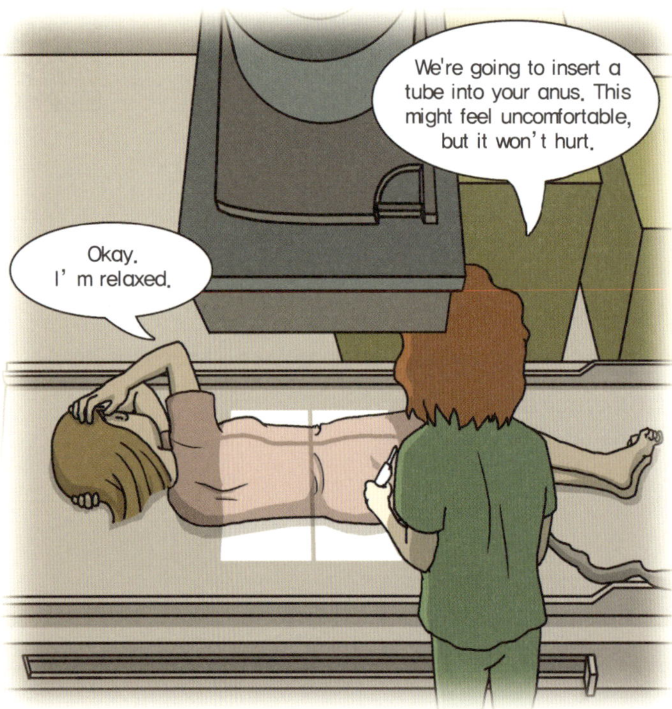

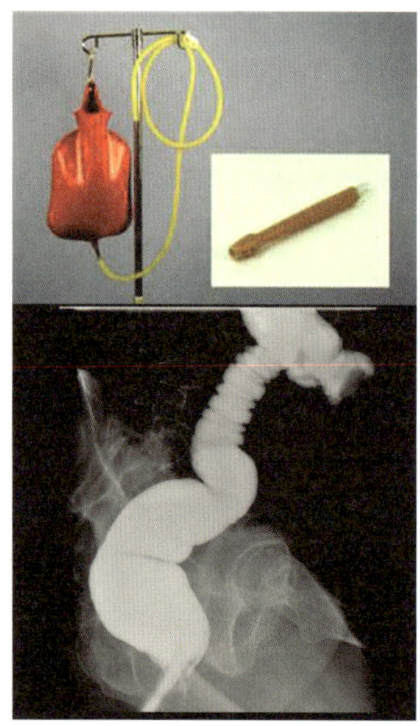

SITUATION ❷

Radiographer Let me aid you in releasing the barium. Please straighten your knees and stand firmly on the board.

Radiographer Next, we'll continue to introduce some air to expand your bowels, which may cause slight abdominal swelling. Squeeze your buttocks together, and if you feel uncomfortable, please let us know.

Patient Okay.

Radiographer Now, lie on your stomach and turn onto your right side, then onto your back. Make two 360-degree turns.

Radiographer This helps ensure an even distribution of the barium in your bowels.

Patient Okay.

Radiographer I will remove the tube now. Please squeeze your buttocks together.

Radiographer Lie on your back, and turn slightly onto your left side.

Radiographer We'll proceed with the X-rays. Just follow the radiologist's instructions.

Patient Of course.

(After the examination)

Radiographer The examination is finished. Do you have any other tests scheduled for today?

Patient No, I believe this is the last one. Can I eat now?

Radiographer Yes, you can. Please drink plenty of water and follow up with your doctor regarding your results.

Patient Thank you so much.

Radiographer When you use the restroom, don't be alarmed if your stool color is white. This is due to the barium and is entirely normal.

Patient Thank you for explaining everything.

* appendix operation : 충수돌기 수술, 맹장수술, * tube : 기구, 삽입관, * sphincter : 항문, 괄약근,
* straighten : 똑바로 펴다., * stand firmly : 똑바로 다리에 힘주어 서기, * swell : 부풀어 오르다.,
* clinch your buttocks tight : 엉덩이에 힘을 주고 단단히 고정하다., * distribute : 골고루 퍼뜨리다.,
* squeeze your bottom tight : 아랫배에 힘을 주다., * what a relief! : 이제 살 것 같네!

B Reviewing Useful Expressions

1 Did you follow the provided instructions?

2 Have you ever had your appendix removed?

3 Please remove your shoes and get onto the examination table.

4 Now, relax your anal muscles. We're going to insert a tube into your anus.

5 I'm now going to pump barium through the inserted tube. Tighten your anal muscles so the Barium doesn't leak.

6 Please straighten your knees and stand firmly on the board.

7 If you feel uncomfortable, please let us know.

8 We're done with the tube now. Please squeeze your buttocks together.

9 When you use the restroom, don't be alarmed if your stool color is white. This is due to the barium and is entirely normal.

C Role playing

상황 ❶

(검사 시행 전)

방사선사 아침 식사를 하셨나요?

환자 아니요. 저는 먹지 말라고 해서 아무것도 먹지 않았습니다.

방사선사 탈의실로 가서 하의를 벗으시고 검사 가운으로 갈아입으세요. 그리고 목걸이와 몸에 있는 모든 금속 물질을 제거하는 것을 잊지 마세요.

환자 예. 알겠습니다.

(환자가 검사실로 들어온다.)

의사 환자분에게 드린 전처치를 지시대로 하셨나요?

환자 예

의사 위장수술이나 맹장수술을 받으신 적이 있나요?

환자 아니요.

의사 신발을 벗으시고 검사 테이블로 올라오세요. 환자분 왼쪽으로 돌아서세요.

환자 예. 알겠습니다.

의사 자, 이제 긴장을 푸세요. 제가 당신의 항문으로 튜브를 넣겠습니다. 좀 불편한 느낌이 들 수 있지만, 아프진 않을 겁니다.

환자 예. 긴장을 풀었어요.

의사 이제 바륨을 삽입된 튜브를 통해 들어갈 것입니다. 바륨이 새지 않도록 항문 근육을 조여 주세요.

상황 ❷

(검사 시행 중)

의사 환자분이 바륨을 퍼지게 할 수 있도록 해드리겠습니다. 양 무릎을 펴시고 발판 위에 똑바로 힘을 주고 서 주세요.

의사 환자분의 장이 부풀도록 공기를 주입하겠습니다. 환자분 복부가 조금 부풀어 오를 겁니다. 엉덩이에 힘을 주고 단단히 고정하세요. 만일 환자분이 힘드시면, 즉시 저희에게 말씀하세요.

환자 네, 알겠습니다.

의사 환자분 위 부분이 아래로 가도록 누우시고, 오른쪽으로 돌아보시고, 위쪽으로 돌아보세요. 360도로 두 번 돌아보세요.

의사 이렇게 하면 바륨이 환자분 장에 골고루 퍼지게 됩니다.

환자 네

의사 자 이제 관을 제거하겠습니다. 환자분 엉덩이를 단단히 조여 주세요.

의사 등을 대고 누우시고, 왼쪽으로 조금 돌아보세요.

의사 자 이제 X선 촬영을 하겠습니다. 방사선사의 지시대로 따라주세요.

환자 물론이지요.

(검사 시행 후)

의사　　검사가 끝났습니다. 또 다른 검사가 있나요?

환자　　아니오. 이 검사가 마지막인것 같아요. 이제 식사를 해도 되나요?

의사　　예. 물을 많이 드시고, 검사 결과는 예약날짜에 담당의사 선생님을 찾아 가시면 됩니다.

환자　　네, 정말 감사합니다.

의사　　화장실을 이용할 때 변 색깔이 하얗다고 해서 놀라지 마세요. 바륨 때문이니 정상입니다.

환자　　설명을 잘해 주셔서 감사합니다.

D Quiz

1 Did you follow the ( ) instructions?

2 I'm now going to ( ) barium through the inserted tube. ( ) your anal muscles so the barium doesn't leak.

3 Let me aid you in releasing the barium. Please ( ) your knees and stand firmly on the board.

4 Now, lie on your stomach and turn onto your right side, then onto your back. Make two 360-degree ( ).

5 I will remove the tube now. Please ( ) your buttocks together.

정답 provided / pump / tighten / straighten / turns / squeeze

E Translate Korean into English

1 환자분 지시대로 약을 드셨나요?

2 자, 이제 긴장을 푸세요. 제가 당신의 항문으로 튜브를 넣겠습니다. 좀 불편한 느낌이 들 수 있지만, 아프진 않을 겁니다.

3 이제 제가 바륨을 넣겠습니다.

4 참으세요. 만일 환자분이 힘드시면, 즉시 저희에게 말씀하세요.

5 이제 식사를 하셔도 됩니다. 물을 많이 드세요.

6 화장실을 이용할 때 변 색깔이 하얗다고 해서 놀라지 마세요. 바륨 때문이니 정상입니다.

Chapter 12

신장조영 검사하기

A Dialogue

SITUATION ❶ I'll be taking a series of X-rays with different positions and time intervals.

Nurse: This is Mrs. Eva Jones, scheduled for an IVP.

Radiographer: Alright, let's head into the examination room.

Radiographer: (for a female patient) Are you married? Do you think you could be pregnant?

Patient: Yes, I'm married. I don't think I am pregnant.

Radiographer: Have you ever had this type of examination before?

Patient: No, this is my first time.

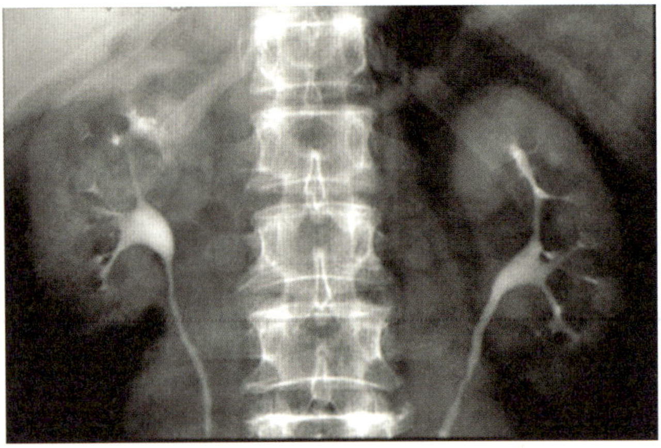

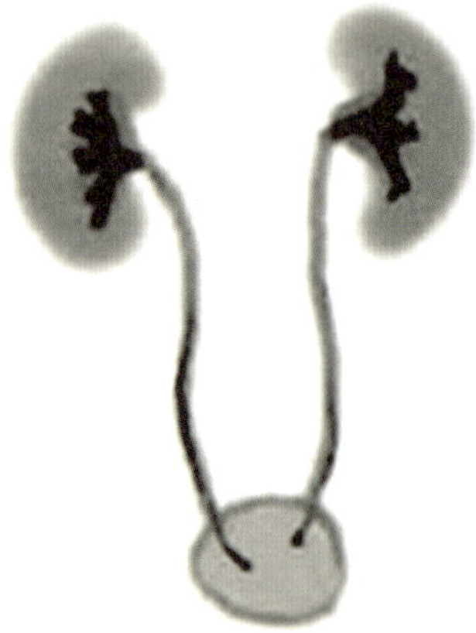

Radiographer	Did your nurse have you fill out an examination agreement?
Patient	Yes.
Radiographer	Do you have any food or medicine allergies?
Patient	No, I don't have any allergies to food or medicine.
Radiographer	Please lie down on the examination table and try to remain still.
Patient	Of course.
Radiographer	Take a deep breath and hold it for a moment. You can breathe normally now.
Radiographer	Ma'am, I'll be injecting a small amount of contrast medium into your IV line as a test dose before giving the full amount.
Patient	That's fine.

Radiographer If you start feeling unwell or experience any abnormal sensations, please let me know immediately.

Patient Yes, I will.

Radiographer Do you feel anything unusual right now, ma'am?

Patient No, I feel fine.

Radiographer I'm now injecting the full dose of the contrast medium. Are you experiencing any discomfort?

Patient I do feel a slight warmth, but it's manageable.

Radiographer If you feel warmth, there's no need to worry; it's a normal sensation.

Radiographer Ma'am, during the procedure, please inform me immediately if you experience itchiness, difficulty in breathing or swallowing, dizziness, or any unusual symptoms. We need to watch out for any signs of allergies.

Patient Yes, I'll definitely let you know if I experience any symptoms.

Radiographer I'll be taking a series of X-rays with different positions and time intervals. Just follow my instructions.

Patient Okay, I will.

* an examination agreement : 검사동의서, * itchiness : 가려움, 좀이 쑤심, * swallowing : 삼키기,
* dizziness : 어지러움

SITUATION ❷

Radiographer The examination is finished. Ma'am, I'll have you wait in the waiting area momentarily and inform the nurse-in-charge. Please be patient while we arrange for your return to your ward.

Patient How long will I have to wait?

Radiographer You will be transferred to your ward as soon as an orderly becomes available.

[Waiting]

Patient I've been waiting here for about 10 minutes. When will I be taken back to my room?

Radiographer I apologize for the delay, ma'am. The orderly has been informed, and they should be here shortly.

Patient I'm getting a bit tired.

Radiographer There was an emergency patient who needed immediate attention, but the orderly will be with you as soon as they finish assisting that patient.

[Waiting]

Orderly I'm here. Where's the patient for transfer?

Radiographer The patient is in the waiting area.

Radiographer Ma'am, I apologize for the wait. The orderly is here now to transfer you back to the ward.

Orderly Ma'am, I'm ready to transfer you now. I'm sorry for the delay; I had to assist an emergency patient first.

Patient It's okay. I understand. Thank you for all of your assistance.

* the orderly : 환자 운반 도우미, 병원의 잡역부, * the ward : 병동, 입원실

B Reviewing Useful Expressions

1 Have you ever had this type of examination before?

2 I'll be taking a series of X-rays with different positions and time intervals. Just follow my instructions.

3 I'll have you wait in the waiting area momentarily and inform the nurse-in-charge.

4 Please be patient while we arrange for your return to your ward.

5 You will be transferred to your ward as soon as an orderly becomes available.

6 There was an emergency patient who needed immediate attention.

7 The orderly will be with you as soon as they finish assisting that patient.

C Role playing

상황 ❶

(검사 시행 전 검사에 대한 설명하기)

간호사 여기 환자 Eva Jones님을 모시고 왔는데요, IVP 검사가 예약됐어요.

방사선사　네. 검사실 안으로 들어가시지요.

방사선사　(여성 환자에게) 결혼하셨나요? 임신 가능성이 있으신가요?

환자　네 기혼입니다. 임신은 아닙니다.

방사선사　이전에 이런 종류의 검사를 받으신 적이 있나요?

환자　아니오. 이 검사는 처음입니다.

방사선사　담당 간호사가 환자분이 검사 동의서를 작성하도록 하셨나요?

환자　예 작성하였습니다.

방사선사　어떤 음식이나 약물에 대해 알레르기를 가지고 계신가요?

환자　아니오. 저는 음식이나 약물에 대해 알레르기가 없습니다.

(검사 시행 중)

방사선사　검사 테이블에 누어보세요. 움직이지 마세요.

환자　알겠습니다.

방사선사　숨을 크게 들여마시고, 숨을 멈추세요. 이제 숨을 쉬어도 됩니다.

방사선사　환자분, 제가 조영제 약물 전량을 투여하기 전에 테스트용으로 약간을 수액 라인을 통해 주입하겠습니다.

환자　좋습니다.

방사선사　만일 기분이 안 좋거나 이상한 느낌이 들면, 즉시 제게 알려주세요.

환자　네, 그렇게 할께요.

(조영제 반응검사 후)

방사선사　환자분, 어떤 이상한 점이라도 느껴지나요?

환자 아니오. 괜찮아요.

방사선사 이제 조영제 전량을 투여하겠습니다. 어떤 불편한 점이라도 느껴집니까?

환자 약간 따뜻한 느낌이 드는데요, 그러나 견딜만합니다.

방사선사 만일 따뜻한 느낌이 든다면, 걱정마세요. 그건 정상입니다.

방사선사 환자분, 제가 이 검사를 하는 동안, 만일 환자분에게 가려움증이나 호흡, 삼키는데 어려움, 어지러움증 혹은 느끼시기에 이상한 증세가 있다면 즉시 저희에게 알려주세요. 저희는 알레르기 반응을 계속 관찰해야 합니다.

환자 네, 알겠습니다. 증상이 있으면 바로 말씀드릴께요.

방사선사 제가 시간 간격을 두고 다른 자세에서 몇 장의 X선 사진을 촬영하겠습니다. 제 지시대로 따라주시기만 하면 됩니다.

환자 예. 잘 알겠습니다.

상황 ❷

(검사 시행 후)

방사선사 검사가 끝났습니다. 환자분, 잠시 대기실에서 기다리시고 담당 간호사님께 알려드리겠습니다. 병동으로 돌아가실 수 있도록 준비하는 동안 잠시만 기다려주세요.

환자 얼마나 기다려야 하나요?

방사선사 순서가 잡혀지는 대로 환자분을 병실로 모시고 갈겁니다.

(대기실에서)

환자 제가 10분 가량 기다리고 있는데요. 언제쯤 내 병실로 돌아갈 수 있나요?

방사선사 환자분, 기다리게 해드려 죄송합니다. 순서대로 직원에게 연락이 왔고 곧 도착할 것입니다.

환자　제가 좀 피곤합니다.

방사선사　즉각적인 치료가 필요한 응급환자가 있었던 것 같아요. 그 환자 보조가 끝나는 대로 직원이 올겁니다.

(잠시 후 환자 이송반 직원이 도착한다.)

환자 이송반 직원　제가 왔습니다. 모시고 갈 환자는 어디 있나요?

방사선사　대기실에 있습니다.

방사선사　환자분 기다리게 해서 죄송합니다. 환자분을 입원실로 모시고 갈 환자 이송반 직원이 왔습니다.

환자 이송반 직원　환자분 제가 환자분을 모시고 가겠습니다. 늦어서 죄송합니다. 환자분에게 오기 전에 우선 응급환자를 돌보았습니다.

환자　괜찮아요. 이해합니다. 여러분 모두에게 감사합니다.

D Quiz

1 Did your (　　　　) have you fill out an examination agreement?

2 I'm now injecting the full dose of the contrast medium. Are you experiencing any (　　　　)?

3 Do you feel anything (　　　　) right now, ma'am?

4 I do feel a slight warmth, but it's (　　　　).

5 You will be transferred to your ward as soon as an orderly becomes (　　　　).

정답　nurse / discomfort / unusual / manageable / available

E Translate Korean into English

1 결혼하셨나요? 임신 가능성이 있으신 가요?

2 만일 환자분에게 가려움증이나 호흡, 삼키는데 어려움, 어지러움증 혹은 느끼시기에 이상한 증세가 있다면 즉시 저희에게 알려주세요.

3 제가 시간 간격을 두고 다른 자세에서 몇 장의 X선 사진을 촬영하겠습니다.

4 환자분이 입원실로 모시고 갈 환자 이송반 직원을 기다려 주세요.

5 환자분 기다리게 해서 죄송합니다. 환자분을 입원실로 모시고 갈 환자 이송반 직원이 왔습니다.

Chapter 13.1

초음파 검사 예약하기

A Dialogue

SITUATION 1 I'll give you instructions and an appointment slip.

Radiographer Good morning, how can I assist you today?

Patient Yes, I'm here for an ultrasound.

Radiographer Do you have a request slip, ma'am?

Patient Ah, yes, here it is.

Radiographer Your name is Lily Johnson, and you are scheduled for an upper abdominal ultrasound.

Patient Yes, that's correct.

Radiographer Ma'am, I need to verify the schedule since this procedure requires some preparation.

Patient Is it possible to schedule it for tomorrow?

Radiographer Let me check... Ah, yes, ma'am, tomorrow at 9 a.m. Does that work for you?

Patient Yes, I'm available at that time.

Radiographer I'll provide you with instructions and an appointment slip.

Patient Sure.

Radiographer Your appointment is tomorrow, Thursday, September 20, at 9 a.m. Here are the instructions for the examination.

Patient Can I take a look at the instructions?

Radiographer Of course. Please have a light dinner and refrain from eating or drinking after midnight. Avoid foods that may produce gas, like beans and carbonated drinks.

Patient Is there anything else I need to do?

Radiographer Yes, if you are a smoker, it's best not to smoke for 12 hours before the appointment. Please return here tomorrow, arriving about five minutes before the scheduled time.

Patient Okay, I understand.

Radiographer If you have any questions, ma'am, you can reach us at this number: 031-740-4312.

Patient Well then, see you tomorrow. Thank you.

Radiographer You're welcome, ma'am.

* beans : 콩류, * carbonated drinks : 탄산음료

B Reviewing Useful Expressions

1 I need to verify the schedule since this procedure requires some preparation.

2 Please have a light dinner and refrain from eating or drinking after midnight.

3 Avoid foods that may produce gas, like beans and carbonated drinks.

4 If you are a smoker, it's best not to smoke for 12 hours before the appointment.

C Role playing

상황 1

방사선사 안녕하세요. 무엇을 도와드릴까요?

환자 예. 저는 초음파검사를 하러 왔습니다.

방사선사 환자분, 검사의뢰서 가지고 계신가요?

환자 아 예, 여기 있습니다. (환자는 방사선사에게 의뢰서를 준다.)

방사선사 환자분 이름은 Lily Johnson 이시고요, 상복부 초음파 검사를 하시네요.

환자 예, 맞습니다.

방사선사 환자분, 이 검사를 하기 위해서는 전처치가 필요하므로 우선 예약 상황을 체크하겠습니다.

환자 제가 내일 검사를 하고자 하는데 가능한가요?

방사선사 한번 봐드릴께요... 아, 예 환자분 내일 오전 9시, 이 시간이면 환자분은 괜찮으신가요?

환자 예. 그 시간이면 가능합니다.

방사선사 제가 환자분에게 지침사항과 예약지를 드리겠습니다.

환자 알겠습니다.

방사선사 환자분의 예약일은 내일, 9월 20일 목요일 오전 9시입니다. 여기 검사에 필요한 지침사항이 있습니다.

환자 그리고 뭐 다른 것도 있나요?

방사선사 저녁에는 부드러운 식사를 하시고 자정 이후에는 아무것도 먹거나 마시면 안 됩니다. 콩류나 탄산음료와 같이 가스를 유발하는 음식은 피해주세요.

환자 제가 해야 할 것이 더 있나요?

방사선사 예, 환자분이 흡연을 하신다면 12시간은 금연하시는 것이 좋습니다. 그러면 내일 환자분의 예약 시간 5분전에 이곳으로 와 주세요.

환자 예, 알겠습니다.

방사선사 만일 환자분이 의문사항이 있으시면 이 전화번호 031-740-4312로 연락주세요.

환자 자, 그럼 내일 뵙겠습니다. 감사합니다.

방사선사 천만에요.

D Quiz

1 Let me check... Ah, yes, ma'am, tomorrow at 9 a.m. Does that (   ) for you?

2 Yes, I'm available (   ) that time.

3 (   ) foods that may produce gas, like beans and carbonated drinks.

4 If you are a smoker, it's (   ) not to smoke for 12 hours before the appointment.

5 If you have any questions, ma'am, you can (   ) us at this number: 031-740-4312.

정답 reach / best / avoid / at / work

E Translate Korean into English

1 환자분 이름은 Lily Johnson 이시고요, 상복부 초음파 검사를 하시네요.

2 저녁에는 부드러운 식사를 하시고 자정 이후에는 아무것도 먹거나 마시면 안 됩니다.

3 콩류나 탄산음료와 같이 가스를 유발하는 음식은 피해주세요.

4 환자분이 흡연을 하신다면 12시간은 금연하시는 것이 좋습니다.

Chapter 13.2

상복부 초음파 검사하기

A Dialogue

SITUATION 1 I'll apply some gel to your tummy.

Patient	Good morning. I have an ultrasound scheduled for today.
Receptionist	Good morning. May I have your appointment slip, ma'am?
Patient	Here it is.
Receptionist	Ma'am, did you follow the instructions provided to you? When did you last eat?
Patient	Yes, I had dinner at 8 p.m., and I haven't had anything since. Now I'm feeling hungry.
Receptionist	That's perfectly fine, ma'am. The procedure won't take too long, and you can eat afterward.
Patient	Thank you.

Receptionist	Please have a seat while I pass your request slip to the radiographer on duty.
Receptionist to Radiographer	You have a request here for an upper abdominal ultrasound. The patient's last meal was at 8 p.m. Her name is Lily Johnson.
Radiographer	Thank you. Are you Lily Johnson?
Patient	Yes, that's me.
Radiographer	Please come into this room, ma'am. I will conduct the scanning.
Patient	Okay, should I remove my jewelry or clothing?
Radiographer	No, ma'am. Just lie down on this bed, raise your hands with your palms resting behind your head, and relax.
Patient	Alright.
Radiographer	I will lift your blouse up and place this blanket over your lower abdomen. I'll apply some gel onto your tummy; it might feel a bit cold. Then I'll start scanning.
Patient	Okay.
Radiographer	Ma'am, take a deep breath and hold it... Alright, you can breathe normally now. Just relax.
Patient	Okay.

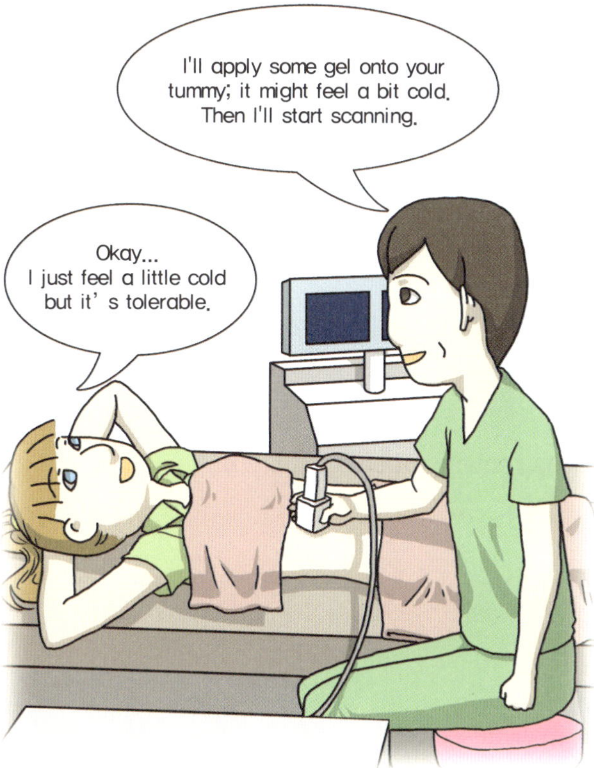

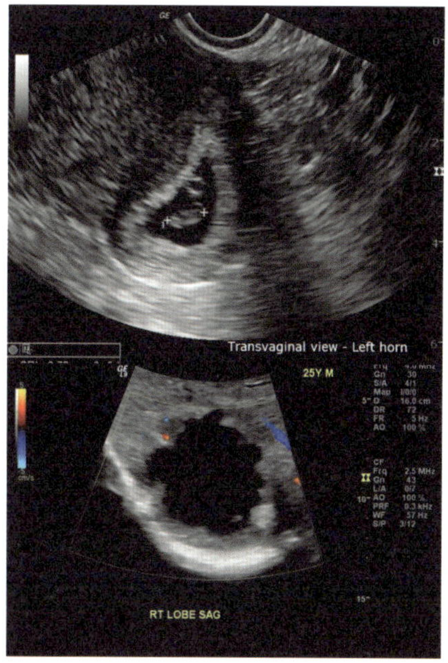

Radiographer If you could kindly turn onto your left side and take a deep breath once more. Hold your breath for a moment... Great, now relax. Now, please turn onto your right side.

Patient Sure.

Radiographer Now, if you could return to lying flat on your back, please. The scan is finished, ma'am.

Radiographer Here are some extra tissues for you to wipe off the gel.

Patient When can I expect the results?

Radiographer Well, ma'am, you can grab a meal first, and then return for the results. The doctor will review the images, and the official results will be ready once they're done. You can pick them up at the reception area and take them to your doctor.

Patient Alright, I'll grab a bite before because I'm quite hungry now. What time does your section close?

Radiographer Ma'am, the reception area remains open until 6 p.m.

Patient Okay, thank you.

Radiographer You're welcome.

[At the reception area]

Patient I'd like to obtain the results of my ultrasound. My name is Lily Johnson.

Receptionist Here are the official results. Please take this to your attending doctor and the doctor will explain the results to you.

Patient Thank you.

Receptionist My pleasure, ma'am.

* tummy : 배

B Reviewing Useful Expressions

1 Ma'am, did you follow the instructions provided to you? When did you last eat?

2 Just lie down on this bed, raise your hands with your palms resting behind your head, and relax.

3 I will lift your blouse up and place this blanket over your lower abdomen.

4 I'll apply some gel to your tummy; it might be a bit cold.

5 Ma'am, take a deep breath and hold it... Alright, you can breathe normally now. Just relax.

6 If you could kindly turn onto your left side and take a deep breath once more. Hold your breath for a moment... Great, now relax. Now, please turn onto your right side.

7 Now, if you could return to lying flat on your back, please.

8 You can pick them up at the reception area and take them to your doctor.

9 Here are some extra tissues for you to wipe off the gel.

C Role playing

상황 1

환자 안녕하세요. 제가 오늘 초음파검사 예약이 되어 있는데요.

접수 안녕하세요? 환자분 예약지를 주시겠어요?

환자 여기 있습니다.

접수	환자분에게 드린 지침사항 대로 하셨나요? 환자분의 마지막 식사는 언제였나요?
환자	예 어제 오후 8시에 저녁을 먹었는데, 그 이후에는 아무것도 먹지 않았습니다. 지금 배가 고파요.
접수	잘하셨어요. 검사는 그리 길지 않을 겁니다. 그리고 검사 후에 식사하실 수 있어요.
환자	감사합니다.
접수	제가 담당 방사선사에게 이 의뢰서를 갖다 드릴동안 앉아계세요.
접수 담당자가 방사선사에게	상복부초음파 검사를 해야 할 의뢰서가 여기 있습니다. 마지막 식사는 오후 8시에 하셨답니다.
방사선사	Lily Johnson님!
환자	예 접니다.
방사선사	환자분 이쪽 방 안으로 들어오세요. 제가 검사를 할 겁니다.
환자	예, 제가 장신구나 옷을 벗어야 하나요?
방사선사	아니오. 이 침대에 누우시기만 하면 됩니다, 똑바로, 환자분 손을 위로 올려주시고, 손바닥을 머리 뒤로 하세요.
환자	예
방사선사	제가 환자분 상의를 올린 다음 이 담요로 환자분 하복부를 덮어 드리겠습니다. 환자분 제가 배위에 젤을 바를 텐데, 좀 차갑습니다. 이제 검사를 시작합니다.
환자	네 알겠습니다.
방사선사	환자분, 심호흡을 해보시고 그리고 그대로 멈추세요... 좋습니다, 이제 숨을 시세요. 긴장을 푸세요.
환자	알겠습니다.

방사선사　좋습니다. 환자분, 환자분 왼쪽으로 돌아보세요. 다시 깊게 호흡하시고 그대로 멈추세요. 자, 환자분 호흡을 유지하시고, 긴장을 푸세요. 그리고 오른쪽으로 돌아보세요.

환자　알겠습니다.

방사선사　자 누운 자세로 돌아오시고, 다시 똑바로 누우세요. 환자분 이제 검사가 끝났습니다.

(방사선사가 환자의 겔을 닦아낸다.)

방사선사　여기 휴지가 더 있으니 젤을 닦아내세요.

환자　언제 결과를 볼 수 있나요?

방사선사　환자분 우선 식사를 하시고 결과를 보러 돌아오세요. 의사 선생님이 바로 사진을 판독하시면 정식 결과가 곧바로 나올 겁니다. 환자분은 접수창구에서 그 결과를 찾으신 다음 환자분의 담당 의사선생님에게 가져다 드리세요.

환자　알겠습니다. 저는 지금 너무 배가 고파서 간단히 식사를 하고 올께요. 이 부서는 몇 시까지 근무를 하시나요?

방사선사　환자분, 접수창구는 오후 6시까지 근무합니다.

환자　예, 감사합니다.

방사선사　천만에요.

(접수창구)

환자　저의 초음파 검사 결과를 찾으러 왔는데요. 제 이름은 Lily Johnson입니다.

접수　환자분 여기 정식 결과가 나왔습니다. 환자분 담당 선생님에게 가져다 드리면 결과를 설명해 주실 겁니다.

환자　예. 감사합니다.

접수　천만에요 환자분.

D Quiz

1 I will (   ) your blouse up and place this blanket over your lower abdomen.

2 I'll (   ) some gel to your tummy.

3 Ma'am, (   ) a deep breath and (   ) it... Alright, you can breathe normally now. Just relax.

정답 hold / take / apply / lift

E Translate Korean into English

1 환자분, 예약지를 주시겠어요?

2 환자분의 마지막 식사는 언제였나요?

3 환자분, 손을 위로 올려주시고 손바닥을 머리 뒤로 하세요.

4 환자분, 심호흡을 해보시고, 그리고 그대로 멈추세요.

5 여기 휴지가 있으니 겔을 닦아내세요.

Chapter 13.3

하복부 초음파 검사하기

A Dialogue

SITUATION ① Before we can proceed with the scanning, you'll need to have a full bladder.

Radiographer Patient Anna Steven.

Patient Yes, I'm here.

Radiographer Ma'am, you're here for a pelvic ultrasound. Before you can proceed with the scanning, you need to have a full bladder. Do you currently feel like using the restroom?

Patient No, not at the moment. I used the restroom before coming here.

Radiographer Alright, then. Please drink four large cups of water or some clear, non-carbonated drink. We need to wait until you have a full bladder.

Patient Okay. Got it.

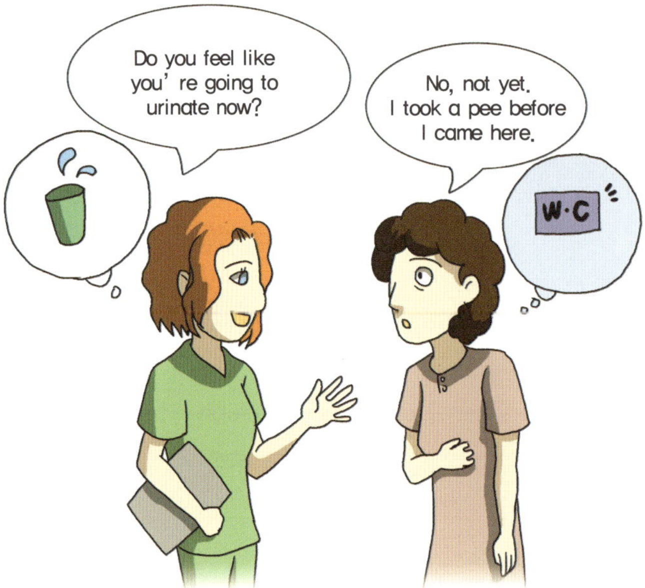
Do you feel like you' re going to urinate now?
No, not yet. I took a pee before I came here.
W·C

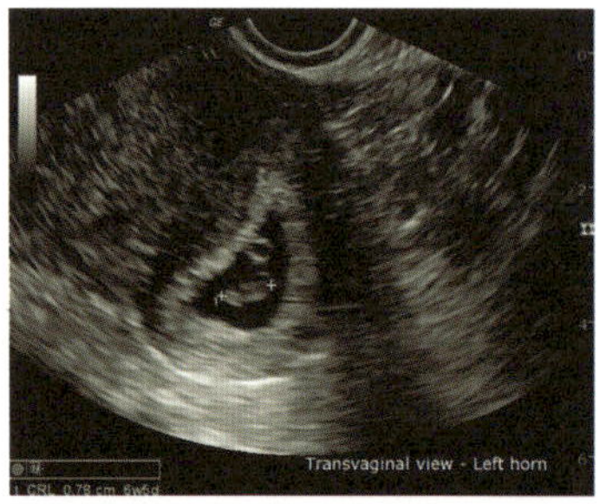

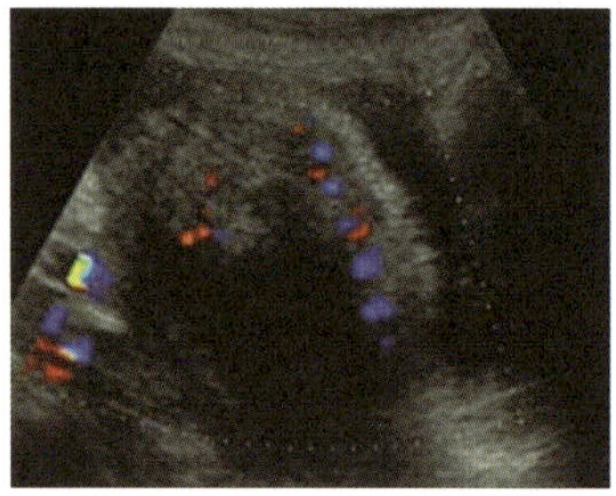

Radiographer	Once you feel an urge to urinate, please let me know immediately. Remember not to use the restroom until your examination is finished.
Patient	Okay.
Radiographer	By the way, ma'am, whenwasthefirstdayofyourlastperiod?
Patient	Oh, thank you. I really need to go.
Patient	I believe it was on May 5th, which was about two weeks ago.
Radiographer	Okay, ma'am. Just let me know right away when you feel the need to use a restroom and we will begin your examination.
Patient	Certainly.

Patient	Miss, I feel like I'm going to need to use the restroom soon.
Radiographer	Alright, ma'am, please come inside.
Patient	Do I need to take off my pants?
Radiographer	No, ma'am, just lie down straight on the bed and place your hands behind your head to relax.
Patient	Okay.
Radiographer	I'll just lower your pants slightly and cover your lower pelvis and legs with a blanket. Then, I'll apply some gel to your lower abdomen and begin the scanning. The gel may feel a bit cold.
Patient	Alright.
Radiographer	Ma'am, the scanning is now complete. You can now use the restroom.

* the urge of urinating : 소변이 심하게 마려움

B Reviewing Useful Expressions

1 Before you can proceed with the scanning, you'll need to have a full bladder.

2 Please drink four large cups of water or some clear, non-carbonated drink. We need to wait until you have a full bladder.

3 Once you feel an urge to urinate, please let me know immediately.

4 Remember not to use the restroom until your examination is finished.

5 Just let me know right away when you feel the need to use the restroom and we will begin your examination.

6 When was the first day of your last period?

C Role playing

방사선사 Anna Steven님.

환자 예, 저 여기 있습니다.

방사선사 환자분은 하복부 초음파검사를 하실 겁니다. 우선 환자분은 검사를 하기 전에 방광을 채우셔야 할 필요가 있습니다. 지금 소변을 보고 싶으신가요?

환자 아니오, 아직은요. 여기 오기 전에 화장실을 다녀왔어요.

방사선사 그러면 알겠습니다. 이제 생수나 비탄산 음료를 큰 컵으로 4번 드세요. 저희는 환자분의 방광이 찰 때까지 기다리겠습니다.

환자 알겠습니다.

방사선사 소변이 몹시 마려우면, 일단 즉시 저에게 말하세요. 소변을 보시면 안 됩니다. 제가 검사하는 동안 환자분의 소변은 그대로 유지해야 합니다.

환자 예 알겠습니다.

방사선사 그런데 환자분, 환자분의 마지막 생리가 시작된 첫날은 언제였나요?

환자 아마 지난 5월 5일인데, 약 2주전 일겁니다.

방사선사 알겠습니다. 환자분. 환자분이 소변이 마려우면 즉시 저에게 알려주세요. 제가 환자분의 검사를 끝내기 전 까지는 소변을 보시면 안 된다는 것을 기억하세요.

환자 물론입니다.

(환자는 물을 마시고 돌아온다.)

환자 선생님, 제가 곧 화장실을 가야할 것 같아요.

방사선사 예 환자분. 안으로 들어오세요.

환자 바지를 갈아입어야 하나요?

방사선사 아닙니다. 침대에 똑바로 누우세요, 두 손을 올리시고, 손바닥을 머리 뒤로 놓으시고, 긴장을 푸세요.

환자 알겠습니다.

방사선사 제가 환자분 바지를 살짝 내리고 골반과 다리를 담요로 덮어드릴께요. 그리고 제가 하복부에 젤을 바르고 나서 검사를 시작하겠습니다. 젤이 좀 차갑습니다.

환자 괜찮습니다.

(방사선사가 검사를 시작한다.)

방사선사 환자분, 검사가 끝났습니다. 화장실에 가셔서 소변을 보세요.

환자 오. 감사합니다. 정말 화장실에 가야할 것 같아요.

D Quiz

1 Ma'am, you're here for a pelvic ultrasound. Before you can proceed with the scanning, you'll need to have a (   ) bladder.

2 Please drink four (   ) of water or some clear, non-carbonated drink.

3 I (   ) the restroom before coming here.

4 Just lie down straight on the bed and (   ) your hands (   ) your head to relax.

5 I'll just (   ) your pants slightly and cover your lower pelvis and legs with a blanket. Then, I'll (   ) some gel to your lower abdomen and begin the scanning.

정답 full / large cups / used / place / behind / lower / apply

E Translate Korean into English

1 우선 환자분은 검사를 하기 전에 방광을 채우셔야 할 필요가 있습니다.

2 투명한 음료나 비탄산 음료를 큰 컵으로 4번 드세요.

3 소변이 심하게 마려우면, 일단 즉시 저에게 말하세요. 소변을 보시면 안 됩니다.

4 두 손을 올리시고, 손을 머리 뒤로 놓으시고, 긴장 푸세요.

5 검사가 끝났습니다. 화장실에 가셔서 소변을 보세요.

Chapter 14

핵의학 검사하기

A Dialogue

SITUATION 1 When you use the restroom, exercise caution to prevent any contact between your urine and your skin or clothing.

Patient Good morning. I'm here for a Bone Scan. My doctor scheduled an appointment for me today.

Radiographer Good morning, sir. Let me check. Did you bring your referral letter?

Patient Yes, here it is.

Radiographer Your name is Nathan Carter.

Patient Yes, that's correct.

Radiographer Sir, please fill out this information sheet and sign the consent form. Make sure to read the attached instructions. Afterward, I'll administer a radiopharmaceutical.

Patient Alright.

Patient I've completed these forms and signed the consent form.

Radiographer I'm going to administer the radiopharmaceutical. You might feel a slight pinch from the needle, but it's bearable.

Patient Are there any side effects?

Radiographer There are no known side effects, so no need to worry.

Patient Okay.

Radiographer Sir, we'll wait for about 4 hours for the radiopharmaceutical to be absorbed before I take the images. You can stay here in the waiting area and watch TV while we wait.

Patient Sounds good.

Radiographer Make sure to drink enough water and use the restroom before we begin scanning. However, when you use the restroom, exercise caution to prevent any contact between your urine and your skin or clothing.

Patient Okay, I understand.

Radiographer Before the examination, change into a hospital gown after using the restroom and remove all your jewelry, accessories, and eyeglasses. You can store all of your belongings in a locker inside the dressing room.

Patient Okay.

SITUATION ❷

Radiographer Sir, I'm going to start the scan. Did you use the restroom before coming in?

Patient Yes, I did.

Radiographer Please lie down on the examination table. Try not to move during the scan; it will only take about 10 to 15 minutes. Just relax.

Patient Sure.

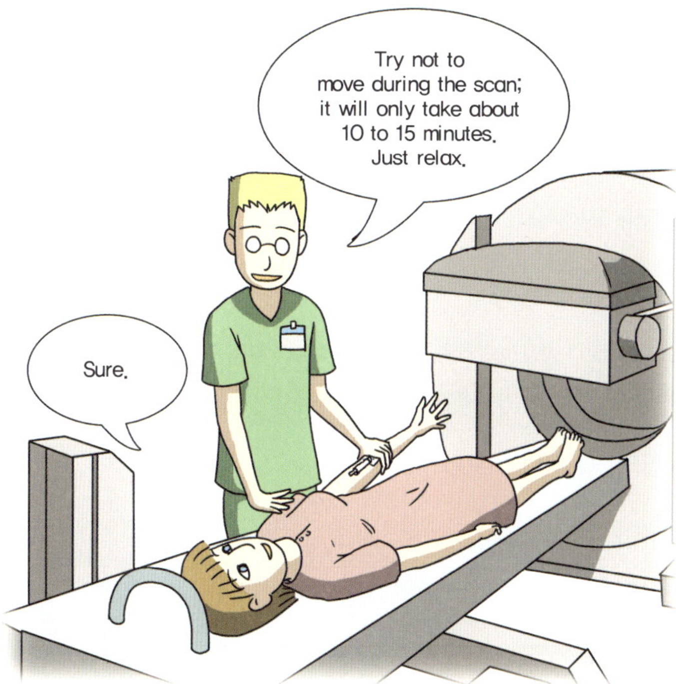

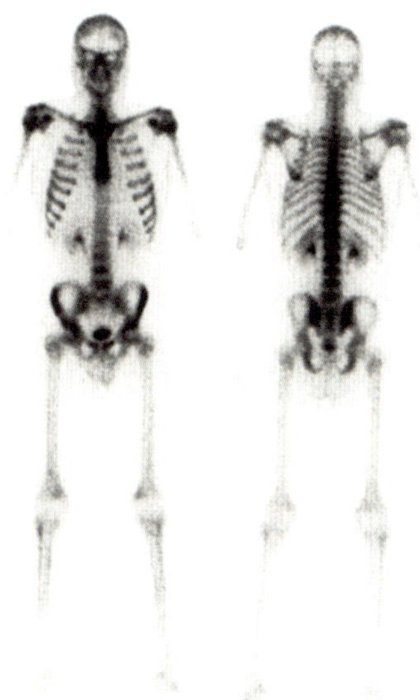

Radiographer The examination is now finished.

Patient When can I expect to receive the results?

Radiographer We'll send the results to your doctor, and you can discuss them at your next appointment with the doctor.

Patient What about the medication you administered? How long will it stay in my system? Can I drive?

Radiographer It won't make you drowsy, so you'll be fine to drive. You can go back to your regular activities. Just remember to drink enough fluids and use the restroom frequently when you get home.

Patient Got it.

Radiographer After about 36 hours, your body will have eliminated the radiopharmaceutical. No need to worry about it.

Patient Alright, thank you.

Radiographer You're welcome, sir.

* bone scan : 뼈검사, * radiopharmaceutical : 방사성의약품, * side effect : 부작용, * drowsiness : 졸음, * resume : 회복하다. 돌아가다., * eliminate : 사라지다. 없어지다.

B Reviewing Useful Expressions

1 I'm going to administer the radiopharmaceutical. You might feel a slight pinch from the needle, but it's bearable.

2 There are no known side effects, so no need to worry.

3 We'll wait for about 4 hours for the radiopharmaceutical to be absorbed before

I take the images.

4 Make sure to drink enough water and use the restroom before we begin scanning. However, when you use the restroom, exercise caution to prevent any contact between your urine and your skin or clothing.

5 Change into a hospital gown after using the restroom and remove all your jewelry, accessories, and eyeglasses.

6 Try not to move during the scan; it will only take about 10 to 15 minutes.

7 Just remember to drink enough fluids and use the restroom frequently when you get home.

8 After about 36 hours, your body will have eliminated the radiopharmaceutical. No need to worry about it.

C Role playing

상황 1

환자 안녕하세요. 뼈검사를 하러 왔어요. 제 담당 의사선생님께서 오늘 이 곳에 저의 검사를 예약을 하셨다고 알고 있습니다.

방사선사 안녕하세요. 환자분. 한번 알아볼께요. 검사의뢰서를 가져오셨나요?

환자 예 여기 있습니다.

방사선사 성함이 Nathan Carter이시군요.

환자 예 맞습니다.

방사선사 환자분, 이 안내 용지를 작성해 주시고 검사 동의서에 서명해 주세요. 그 용지에 포함된 지시사항을 읽어주세요. 그 다음에 제가 방사성의약품을 주사하겠습니다.

환자 예 알겠습니다.

환자 저는 이 용지의 내용들을 작성했고 검사 동의서에 이미 서명했습니다.

방사선사 제가 방사성의약품을 주사하겠습니다. 주사바늘이 약간 아프지만 견딜 만합니다.

환자 주사에 부작용이 있나요?

방사선사 지금까지 알려진 부작용은 없습니다. 부작용에 대해 걱정하지 않으셔도 됩니다.

환자 예 알겠습니다.

(방사성의약품 투여 후)

방사선사 환자분, 제가 사진을 촬영하기 전에 방사성의약품이 흡수되어야 하므로 약 4시간 정도 기다리겠습니다. 환자분은 대기실에서 머물러계시고 기다리는 동안 TV를 보고 계셔도 됩니다.

환자 네, 알겠습니다.

방사선사 물을 충분히 드세요. 그리고 검사 전에 소변을 보세요. 그러나 소변을 보실 때, 피부나 옷에 오염되지 않도록 피해주세요.

환자 예 알겠습니다.

방사선사 환자분이 검사하시기 전에, 소변을 보시고 모든 장신구나 손목시계 그리고 안경을 제거해주신 다음 병원 가운으로 갈아입도록 하세요. 환자분의 소지품들은 탈의실 안쪽의 라커에 보관해 주세요.

환자 알겠습니다.

(검사 시행)

상황 ❷

방사선사 환자분, 이제 검사를 시작하겠습니다. 여기 오시기 전에 소변을 보셨나요?

환자 물론입니다.

방사선사 검사테이블에 누워주세요.
검사하는 동안 움직이지 마세요. 이 검사는 10~15분가량 걸립니다. 편하게 계세요.

환자 알겠습니다.

(검사 시행 후)

방사선사 검사가 끝났습니다.

환자 언제 결과를 볼 수 있나요?

방사선사 저희가 결과를 담당 의사선생님께 보내드리겠습니다. 환자분은 진료예약날짜에 담당 의사선생님을 찾아 가시면 됩니다.

환자 선생님이 주사하신 약은 무엇인가요? 그 약은 제 몸 안에 얼마나 오래 남아있게 되나요? 제가 운전을 해도 되나요?

방사선사 그 약은 졸음을 유발시키지 않아요. 환자분은 운전하실 수 있습니다. 환자분은 정상적인 활동을 하실 수 있습니다. 다만 집에 가셔서 수분을 많이 드시고 자주 소변을 보도록 하세요.

환자 예 알겠습니다.

방사선사 약 36시간 후에는 방사성의약품은 환자분 몸에서 사라질 겁니다. 그 점에 대해서는 걱정하지 마세요.

환자 예 감사합니다.

방사선사 천만에요 환자분.

D Quiz

1 Exercise caution to prevent any ( ) between your urine and your skin or clothing.

2 Just remember to drink ( ) fluids and ( ) the restroom frequently when you get home.

3 You can ( ) all of your belongings in a locker inside the dressing room.

4 After about 36 hours, your body will have eliminated the ( ).

정답 radiopharmaceutical / store / use / enough / contact

E Translate Korean into English

1 제가 방사성의약품을 주사하겠습니다. 주사바늘이 약간 아프지만 견딜 만합니다.

2 지금까지 알려진 부작용은 없습니다. 부작용에 대해 걱정하지 않으셔도 됩니다.

3 소변을 보실 때, 피부나 옷에 오염되지 않도록 피해주세요.

4 검사하는 동안 움직이지 마세요. 이 검사는 10~15분가량 걸립니다.

5 약 36시간 후에는 방사성의약품은 환자분 몸에서 사라질 겁니다.

Chapter 15

방사선 치료하기

A Dialogue

SITUATION 1 I need to mark your skin with a tattoo along the treatment area.

Patient	Good morning. I have an appointment for radiation therapy today. My doctor set it up.
Radiographer	Good morning, ma'am. Let me check. Do you have your referral letter with you?
Patient	Yes, here it is.
Radiographer	Your name is Lucy Wilson?
Patient	Yes, that's correct.
Radiographer	Did you follow your doctor's instructions? When was your last meal?
Patient	Yes, my doctor told me not to eat, drink, or take any medication for 6 hours before my appointment. I had a midnight snack, and that was

my last food intake. I haven't had breakfast.

Radiographer Okay, please fill out this information sheet and sign the consent form. Be sure to read the attached instructions.

Patient Alright.

Patient I've completed these forms and signed the consent form.

Radiographer Great. Please go to the dressing room and change into a hospital gown.

Patient Do I need to remove my jewelry and watch?

Radiographer Yes, and you can store your belongings in the locker inside the dressing room.

Patient Okay.

Patient Where should I go next?

Radiographer The doctor will inject a contrast media first, and then I'll guide you to the simulation room.

Patient I'm feeling a bit nervous.

Radiographer Don't worry, ma'am. I'm here to assist you.

Patient Thank you.

Radiographer Please lie down on the table, and I'll adjust your positioning. I'll also be placing an immobilization device on you. It's crucial that you remain still. Just relax.

Patient Okay.

Radiographer Ma'am, I need to mark your skin with a tattoo along the treatment area. Then, I'll be in and out of this room to capture images. But don't worry, we have cameras and intercoms to keep you under constant observation. If you encounter any issues, just let me know.

Patient Sure.

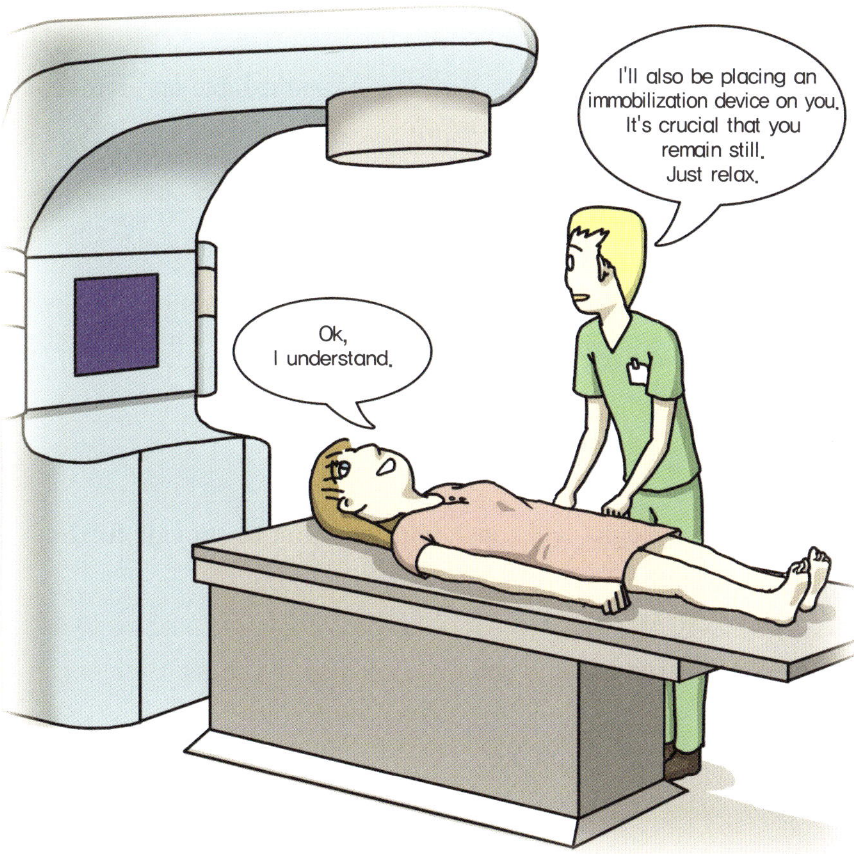

Radiographer	Ma'am, we'll now move to the treatment room.
Patient	I thought we were finished.
Radiographer	We've completed the treatment planning. Now, we have to proceed with the radiation treatment.
Patient	Alright. How long will that take?
Radiographer	It will only take about 20 minutes.
Patient	I see.
Radiographer	Ma'am, please lie down on the treatment table and remain still. Stay calm; it's a similar procedure to earlier, just shorter. If you experience any problems, inform me right away.
Patient	Certainly.
Radiographer	The treatment is finished. How are you feeling, ma'am?
Patient	I feel fine, just a little hungry.
Radiographer	The oncologist will speak with you first to provide further instructions and schedule your follow-up.
Patient	Alright then, thank you.
Radiographer	You're welcome, ma'am.

* simulation room : 시뮬레이션 방, 모의실험 방, * immobilization device : 환자 고정용 장치, * tattoo : 문신, 치료부위 표시, * Oncologist : 종양학 전문의

B Reviewing Useful Expressions

1 The doctor will inject a contrast media first, and then I'll guide you to the simulation room.

2 Don't worry, ma'am. I'm here to assist you.

3 I'll also be placing an immobilization device on you. It's crucial that you remain still. Just relax.

4 Ma'am, I need to mark your skin with a tattoo along the treatment area.

5 Now, we have to proceed with the radiation treatment.

6 It's a similar procedure to earlier, just shorter.

7 The oncologist will speak with you first to provide further instructions and schedule your follow-up.

C Role playing

환자　안녕하세요. 저는 여기에 방사선치료가 예약이 되어 있습니다. 제 담당 의사선생님께서 예약 날짜를 오늘로 잡아두신 것으로 알고 있습니다.

방사선사　안녕하세요. 환자분. 알아보겠습니다. 치료 의뢰서를 가지고 계신가요?

환자　예. 여기 있습니다.

방사선사　성함이 Lucy Wilson이신가요?

환자　예, 맞습니다.

방사선사　담당 의사선생님께서 주신 지시사항을 따르셨나요? 환자분의 마지막 식사는 언제였나요?

환자 예. 제 담당 의사선생님께서는 이곳의 예약 6시간 이전에는 아무것도 먹거나 마시거나 약도 먹지 말라고 하셨습니다. 자정쯤에 간단한 스낵을 먹었습니다. 그 때가 마지막 식사였습니다. 아직 아침은 안 먹었습니다.

방사선사 그럼 됐습니다. 이 안내용지를 작성 하시고 동의서에 서명해 주세요. 그 용지에 포함된 지시사항을 읽어보세요.

환자 알겠습니다. 저는 이미 이들 용지를 작성하였고 동의서에 서명하였습니다.

방사선사 탈의실로 가셔서 입으신 옷을 병원 가운으로 갈아입으세요.

환자 제 악세서리나 손목시계를 빼야 하나요?

방사선사 예. 탈의실 안쪽 라커에 소지품을 보관해 두세요.

환자 알겠습니다.

(환자가 탈의실에서 나온다.)

환자 이제 어디로 가야 하나요?

방사선사 먼저 의사선생님께서 조영제를 주사하실 겁니다. 그 다음 제가 시뮬레이션 방으로 모시고 가겠습니다.

환자 좀 떨리는군요.

방사선사 환자분 걱정하지 마세요. 제가 여기서 환자분을 계속 도와드리겠습니다.

환자 감사합니다.

(검사실로 들어간다.)

방사선사 테이블에 올라가 누우시면 제가 환자분의 자세를 똑바로 잡아드리겠습니다. 제가 고정장치를 부착할 겁니다. 이 장치는 환자분을 움직이지 않도록 하는 중요한 것입니다. 긴장을 푸시면 됩니다.

환자 알겠습니다.

방사선사　환자분, 제가 환자분 치료 부위의 피부에 치료부위 표시를 그리겠습니다. 그 다음 이 방 밖으로 나가서 사진을 촬영하겠습니다. 그렇지만 저희는 환자분을 계속 관찰하기 위해서 카메라와 인터컴으로 보고있습니다. 만일 무슨 문제가 있으면 즉시 저에게 알려주세요.

(검사가 종료됨)

방사선사　환자분, 이제 저희가 치료실로 옮겨드리겠습니다.

환자　저는 끝났는줄 알았어요.

방사선사　저희는 이제 막 치료계획을 끝냈습니다. 이제 방사선 치료를 해야 합니다.

환자　예. 얼마나 걸릴까요?

방사선사　약 20분가량이 소요될 겁니다.

환자　알겠습니다.

방사선사　환자분, 치료테이블에 누워주시고 움직이지 마세요. 그대로 계시고 긴장을 푸세요. 저희가 방금 전에 했던 것과 거의 같은 방법인데 이번은 좀 더 시간이 짧게 걸릴 겁니다. 그래도 환자분이 어떤 문제가 있으시면 즉시 저희에게 알려주세요.

환자　물론이지요.

(치료 시행 후)

방사선사　치료가 끝났습니다. 기분이 어떠세요?

환자　괜찮아요. 그저 좀 허기가 지네요.

방사선사　우선 담당 종양학 전문의께서 환자분에게 어떤 말씀을 해 주실 겁니다. 그분은 환자분에게 앞으로의 지시사항을 알려드리고 추가사항을 말씀 해 주실 겁니다.

환자　예 감사합니다.

방사선사　천만에요. 환자분.

D Quiz

1 Please lie down on the table, and I'll ( ) your positioning. I'll also be placing an ( ) device on you.

2 It's crucial that you ( ) still. Just relax.

3 Ma'am, I need to mark your skin with a ( ) along the treatment area.

4 We've completed the treatment ( ). Now, we have to proceed with the radiation ( ).

정답 adjust / immobilization / remain / tattoo / planning / treatment

E Translate Korean into English

1 환자분 걱정하지마세요. 제가 여기서 환자분을 계속 도와드리겠습니다.

2 제가 고정 장치를 부착할 겁니다. 이 장치는 환자분을 움직이지 않도록 하는 중요한 것입니다.

3 저희는 환자분을 계속 관찰하기 위해서 카메라와 인터컴으로 보고있겠습니다.

4 만일 무슨 문제가 있으면 즉시 저에게 알려주세요.

Chapter 16
취업을 위한 인터뷰하기

A Dialogue

SITUATION 1 I graduated from SG College in 2023.

Interviewer	Welcome to SG Hospital. What motivated you to apply here?
Applicant	I've heard that this is the best place to work.
Interviewer	Do you have any work experience?
Applicant	Yes, I worked as a receptionist at a clinic.
Interviewer	Where did you graduate from?
Applicant	I graduated from SG College in 2023.

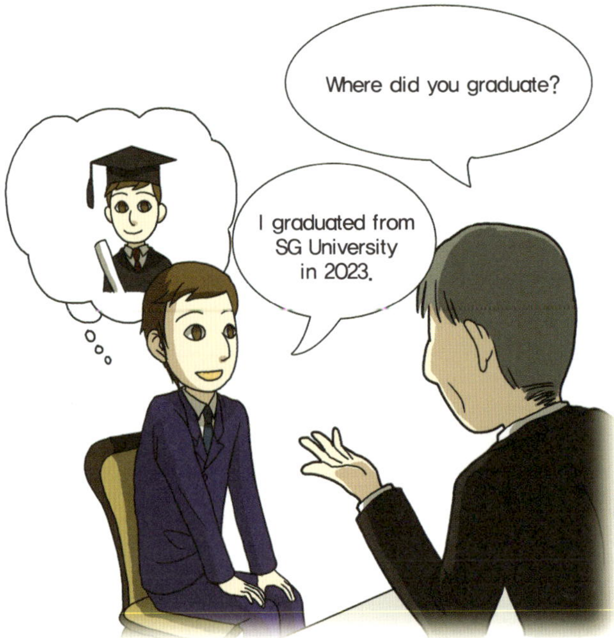
Where did you graduate?
I graduated from SG University in 2023.

Interviewer Any special skills you'd like to mention?

Applicant I'm proficient with computers and have strong interpersonal skills.

Interviewer How would you describe your personality?

Applicant I'm a hardworking and optimistic individual, and I take my responsibilities seriously.

SITUATION ❷ I have a genuine interest in imaging technology, and I enjoy working with patients.

Interviewer Tell me about your educational background.

Applicant I graduated from SG College in 2023 with a degree in Radiological Technology.

Interviewer Why do you want to pursue a career as a Radiographer?

Applicant I have a genuine interest in imaging technology, and I enjoy working with patients.

Interviewer Why should we consider you for this role?

Applicant I believe my educational background would be an asset to your institution.

Interviewer Can you work well with others?

Applicant Yes, I'm friendly and can work well in a team setting.

Interviewer Do you speak any foreign languages?

Applicant Yes, I can speak two foreign languages: English and Chinese.

Interviewer Interesting. Why do you think you're a good fit for this job?

Applicant In addition to my experience, I possess a strong educational background and a strong sense of responsibility.

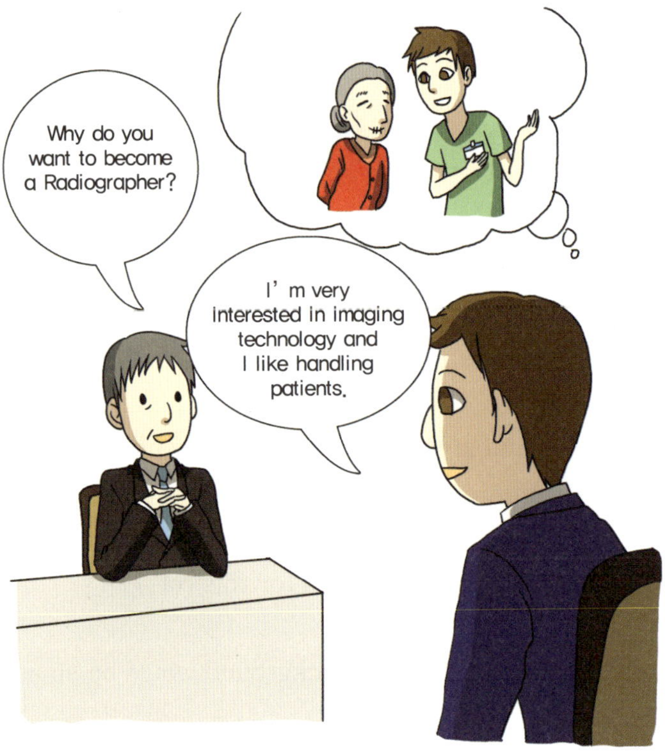
Why do you want to become a Radiographer?
I' m very interested in imaging technology and I like handling patients.

SITUATION 3 I worked for eight months at a diagnostic center.

Interviewer Nice to meet you. I'm the Director of the Personnel Department.

Applicant Nice to meet you too. I'm Jongil Kim, applying for the entry-level Radiographer position.

Interviewer We're specifically looking for someone with related work experience. Do you have any?

Applicant Yes, I worked for 8 months at a diagnostic center.

Interviewer Any specific skills or talents you'd like to highlight?

Applicant I'm fluent in English and Chinese, and I'm proficient with computers.

Interviewer That's great. How do you think you can contribute to our clinic?

Applicant Beyond my skills, I excel in patient care and interpersonal interactions.

Interviewer Can you tell us about your personal qualities?

Applicant I'm hardworking, responsible, and a team player, always ready to collaborate.

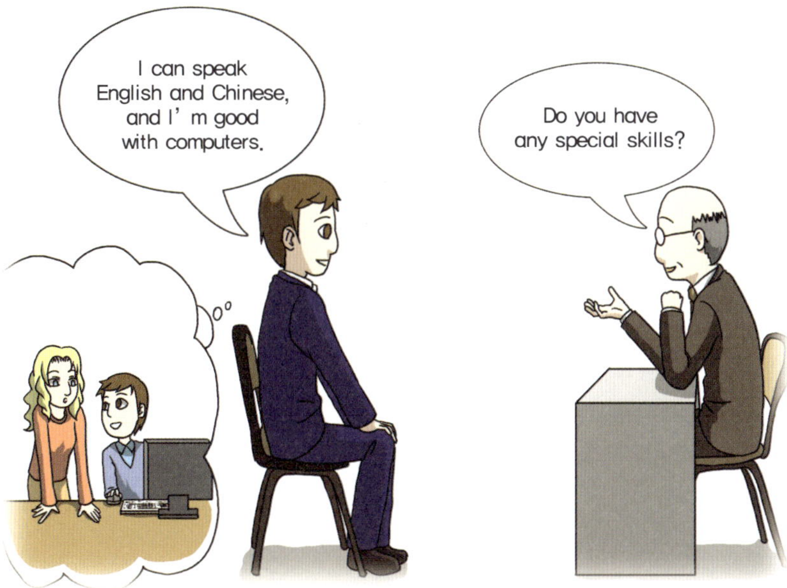
I can speak English and Chinese, and I' m good with computers.
Do you have any special skills?

B Reviewing Useful Expressions

1 Yes, I worked as a receptionist at a clinic.

2 I'm proficient with computers and have strong interpersonal skills.

3 I have a genuine interest in imaging technology, and I enjoy working with patients.

4 Yes, I'm friendly and can work well in a team setting.

5 I've heard that this is the best place to work.

6 I'm hardworking, responsible, and a team player, always ready to collaborate.

C Role playing

상황 ❶ 저는 2023년에 SG 대학교를 졸업하였습니다.

면접관 SG 병원에 오신 것을 환영합니다. 우리 병원에 지원하게 된 동기가 무엇인가요?

응시자 저는 이 곳이 최선을 다해 일하기에 제일 좋은 회사라고 알고 있습니다.

면접관 어떤 경력이라도 있으신가요?

응시자 저는 클리닉에서 접수업무를 해본 적이 있습니다.

면접관 어느 학교를 졸업하셨나요?

응시자 저는 2014년에 SG 대학을 졸업하였습니다.

면접관 어떤 다른 특기라도 가지고 계신가요? 있다면 무엇인가요?

응시자 저는 컴퓨터를 잘 다룰 수 있습니다. 뿐만 아니라 저는 좋은 대인관계를 가지고 있습니다.

면접관 당신의 성격은 어떤지 말해주세요.

응시자 저는 매우 근면하고 낙천적입니다. 그리고 저는 강한 책임감을 가지고 있습니다.

상황 ❷ 저는 방사선 영상기술에 매우 관심이 많고 환자들을 대하며, 일하는 것을 좋아합니다.

면접관 당신의 학력에 대해 말해 주세요.

응시자 저는 2023년도에 SG대학의 방사선학과를 졸업하였습니다.

면접관 왜 당신은 방사선사가 되기로 했나요?

응시자 저는 방사선 영상기술에 매우 관심이 많고, 환자들을 대하며 일하는 것을 좋아합니다.

면접관 당신은 다른 사람들과 어울려 잘 일할 수 있나요?

응시자 네, 저는 친화적이고, 팀 안에서 일을 잘 할 수 있습니다.

면접관 당신은 외국어를 할 수 있나요?

응시자 네, 저는 영어와 중국어, 2가지 외국어를 할 수 있습니다.

면접관 알겠습니다. 당신은 왜 이 일에 적합하다고 생각합니까?

응시자 저의 경험뿐만 아니라 저는 높은 학업능력과 강한 책임감을 가지고 있다고 생각합니다.

상황 ❸ 저는 진단검사센터에서 8개월 동안 근무했습니다.

면접관 만나서 반갑습니다. 저는 인사부장입니다.

응시자 만나서 반갑습니다. 저는 김종길이라고 합니다. 저는 일반 방사선사 직종에 응시하였습니다.

면접관 우리는 이 분야에 경력이 있는 사람을 찾고 있습니다. 당신을 어떤 경력을 가지고 있습니까?

응시자 예, 저는 진단검사센터에서 8개월 동안 근무했습니다.

면접관 다른 특기라도 가지고 있습니까?

응시자 저는 영어와 중국어를 잘 할 수 있으며, 컴퓨터에도 능숙합니다.

면접관 좋습니다. 우리 병원을 위해 무엇을 할 수 있나요?

응시자 저의 전공 분야 뿐만 아니라 저는 환자와 다른 사람 사이의 관계를 원활하게 할 수 있습니다.

면접관 당신의 성격은 어떻습니까?

응시자 저는 매우 근면하고 책임감이 있으며 그리고 협동적입니다. 저는 팀웍을 중요하게 생각합니다.

D Quiz

1 What motivated you to ( ) here?

2 I graduated ( ) SG College in 2023.

3 Tell me about your educational ( ).

4 Why do you want to ( ) a career as a Radiographer?

5 We're specifically ( ) for someone with related work experience.

6 I'm ( ) in English and Chinese, and I'm ( ) with computers.

정답 treatment / planning / tattoo / remain / immobilization / adjust

E Translate Korean into English

1 저는 클리닉에서 접수업무를 해본 적이 있습니다.

2 저는 컴퓨터를 잘 다룰 수 있습니다. 뿐만 아니라 저는 좋은 인간관계 맺는 기술을 가지고 있습니다.

3 저는 다른 사람들과 어울려 일을 잘 하며 매우 우호적입니다.

4 저는 2가지 외국어를 할 수 있습니다.

5 저는 방사선기술학을 전공으로 하였습니다.

6 저는 매우 근면하고 책임감이 있으며, 그리고 팀워크를 중요하게 생각합니다.

REFERENCES

BOOKS

1. 오지은의 메디컬 영어회화(General Hospital Part 1), 청구문화사, 2011.
2. Park Jin Seup, Moon Young Hae. Medical English 3rd edition.

WEBSITES

1. www.memidex.com
2. www.thefreedictionary.com
3. Conversation at Radiology Department (Sourced from Communicating in English-English Conversation for Hospital Workers,published by Health Department, Executive Yuan). lms.ctl.cyut.edu.tw/sys/read_attach.php?id.=179646
4. Bone Scan Division of Nuclear Medicine BWH (Brighan & Women's Hospital) www.brighamandwomens.org/Departments_and_services/radiology services/ nuclear medicine/Patient/bone.aspx
5. http://radiopaedia.org/cases

MEMO

MEMO

MEMO

방사선사를 위한 **병원실무영어**

2013년 3월 8일 초판 발행
2014년 3월 27일 개정판 발행
2024년 2월 28일 개정2판 발행

펴낸이 유광열 · 이주영
삽 화 유수현
발행인 윤진영
발행처 도서출판 대학서림
(110-530) 서울시 종로구 혜화로 2길 8
전 화 02) 763-1220, 744-2812
팩 스 02) 744-1210
등 록 1965. 1. 20
번 호 1-88

정가 18,000원

ISBN 978-89-6940-323-0 13740